MW01138642

Published by Rory Z

1st edition published May 2018

Paperback ISBN: 978-1985818460

Hypno-Fasting is the registered trademark of Rory Z Fulcher and may not be used by any means or in any form whatsoever without written permission.

Author Photograph by Ché Ballard
(www.cheballard.com)

HYPNO®
FASTING

THE SIMPLE, EFFECTIVE WAY TO LOSE WEIGHT BUT STILL EAT ALL THE FOOD YOU LOVE

RORY Z FULCHER

Contents

*Free MP3 Download

Instructions on how to download your copy of the free **Hypno-Fasting** hypnosis MP3 are provided later on in the book. This is because *you need to read the book first, before* listening to the MP3 (it's *much* more effective this way).

Read on, and you'll find the MP3 download exactly where you need it...

About the Author

Rory Z Fulcher is an international hypnotist, therapist, hypnosis trainer and author with many years of experience in the hypnosis industry. He is an avid (amateur) bodybuilder and fitness enthusiast and is also a qualified fitness instructor.

For more information on Rory, please visit his website: **Rory-Z.com**

Other books by Rory Z Fulcher:
The Instant Hypnosis and Rapid Inductions Guidebook (2013)
The Beginner's Guide to Hypnotherapy (2014)
Sam the Sleepy Sheep: The best way to get children to go to sleep (2015)

DVDs by Rory Z Fulcher:
Hypnosis 101: Learn to Hypnotise FAST (2014)
Hypnosis 101: Learn to be a Comedy Hypnotist (2014)

Foreword/Warning

Hello, and welcome to **Hypno-Fasting**! This book may be unlike any book you've ever read before (it's certainly unlike any I've written before).

Purely for entertainment and motivational purposes, this book contains some swearing (not quite a shit-load, but almost), and a whole bunch of straight-talking, advice with no "sugar coating". So, if anything within this book challenges you, or hurts your delicate sensibilities, then good! Occasionally we need to be pushed hard in the right direction, because sometimes 'knowing what we *should* do' doesn't equate to actually doing it. So, I'm here to help give you that push, and to make sure you have a bit of fun whilst you're learning how to easily lose weight! Oh, and while we're on the subject of fun, if you're easily offended or have no sense of humour, you might want to go and buy another diet book... Maybe pick a boring one, written by some smug, teeth-whitening, fake-tanning, overly-PC "health and wellness guru" or something (...and if you do, please make sure to leave an Amazon review for **Hypno-Fasting** telling everyone exactly how it hurt your feelings ...but still feel free to give me 5 stars for being honest from the outset). #ItsTheBestPolicy

This book is for REAL people who want to make REAL changes happen, so it's full of highly effective tips, techniques and information that's easy to digest (no pun intended), but also, equally easy to apply.

This book is *not* filled with scientific mumbo-jumbo (you may have already figured *that* out by the fact that I'm using hashtags in a book... lol), and that's because I'm not here to *bore* the fat off of your ass!

So, before you get started I just thought I'd let you know that this shit is not hard... actually, it's one of the simplest (but most effective) things you'll ever learn to do, and you'll learn to do it easily!

Warning: If you have any current health conditions or concerns (especially hypoglycemia, thyroid problems, diabetes, etc.) or if you are under 18 or over 65 please consult your doctor/physician before putting these methods to use – better safe than sorry.

Also, please do not use the methods presented in this book if:
- You're pregnant/breastfeeding.
- You exercise excessively (i.e. more than 2-3 hours per day).
- You don't get enough sleep.
- You're under massive psychological stress.
- You're using appetite suppressants or fat-loss supplements.
- You're pretending to be healthy to cover up an eating disorder or to drastically control your daily food/calorie intake.

Introduction

If you've read lots of diet books in the past (which, to be fair, most of us who have ever wanted to "lose weight" probably have), then you'll *probably* be used to the introduction chapter being all about how mind-numbingly great the author is. How, since discovering their diet, they've managed to stick to it 24/7/365 without screwing it up. How they *love* eating brussel sprouts, quinoa and other terrible-tasting 'health foods' (mmm hmm, I bet). How they always find time to go out running every day and make it home 90 minutes later, hair still in perfect shape and without even the tiniest bead of sweat on their clean, fluorescent lycra onesie...

Well I'm sick of that crap. That's not me (and I assume it's probably not you either). Personally, I absolutely suck at sticking to diets! I tried a "low carb" diet once and I managed about a month (...a *horrible* month...) before I had a meltdown and immediately drove to the nearest burger restaurant and had 2 double cheeseburgers with extra fries ...for starters. I am *genuinely* not a fan of many so-called "healthy recipes", and doing any cardio-type exercise (running, cycling, swimming, walking up more than one flight of stairs) makes me want to curl up into a ball and die. Sound familiar? If so, I think we're going to be friends! And even if you're *not* like me, even if you *can* stick to diets, *do* like vegetable smoothies and *love* running for miles (seriously, wtf is wrong with you? Jokes, lol), yet you still can't quite shift that extra couple of pounds of fat, well, I think this book might be able to help you too.

Hypno-Fasting is suitable for anyone to read and use, regardless of age, sex, race, activity-level or even your current diet (i.e. the type of food that you eat). Literally almost anybody can benefit from these very simple techniques, with relatively little effort, and no matter what your weight loss requirements are.

You can benefit from these techniques if you usually yo-yo diet or if you've tried lots of different diets and nothing really worked in the long-term. You can lose weight with these techniques if your dieting experience up until this point led you to believe that nothing would ever help you shift the fat. You can *even* succeed at this if you're sceptical about the process itself! Honestly, I was sceptical about the whole 'fasting' thing when I first started doing my research, but then I lost 14lb (6.3kg) of body fat in 4 weeks without changing my diet! That quickly and effectively convinced me that this stuff works, and if it can work for me, it can work for you too.

"OK, I'm psyched! Let's start this diet!"
Awesome, that's the spirit! OK, so the first thing that you're going to want to do is take the word "diet" and completely delete it from your vocabulary. It's time for diets to die. You do not need to "diet" and I am not "putting you on a diet", because diets are

mostly a load of crap. I am not going to ask you to give up all of those tasty things that make you feel great when you shove them into your face-hole. I do not have the slightest desire to make you suffer countless, never-ending glasses of kale-and-spinach smoothies (*vomit*). You shouldn't have to endure skin-crawlingly cold showers, and I am definitely-bloody-not going to recommend that you have a lukewarm coffee enema every Tuesday (seriously, that's a thing – don't believe me? Google it and I bet you'll never think about a cappuccino in the same way again). #Crappuccino

"So, if this book isn't about a diet, then what the hell is it actually about?"
Well like I said; it doesn't really matter *what kind* of food you eat (to a certain degree), but what really does make a huge difference is if you change *when* you eat. Quite simply, you just need to change the timing of your meals. The "eating plans" in this book (that I'm going to teach you to use) have been organised into a process known as "intermittent fasting" ...which sounds more complicated than it is, trust me. Learning to utilise an effective intermittent fasting (IF) plan means you can lose weight whilst continuing to eat all that delicious food that you love!

You don't have to go out and blow your entire pay check buying expensive lean meats or specially tailored "diet meals" and "fat-loss supplements", you won't have to constantly psych yourself up to eat bland, tasteless low-fat options that come in child-sized portions, you don't even need to quit buying all that unhealthy, fatty/sugary crap that probably caused you to be overweight in the first place, if you don't want to...

"What?! You're telling me that just eating at different times will help me lose weight?"
Yes, absolutely! But there's a little more to it than that... Basically, by changing your meal times to fit into a pre-set plan (which I'll explain in a while), your body will have a bit more time with no food available in the stomach. Now as you may or may not know, your body usually uses the food that you put in your stomach as its main source of fuel, which gives you energy to do all the interesting stuff that you do every day (like watching funny videos on YouTube and procrastinating... No? Just me?) So, what happens if there's no food in your stomach to provide you with energy? The energy needs to come from somewhere, so where does it come from?

"I have no idea... what am I, a doctor?"
I thought you might say that. Well, once your super-smart, energy-efficient body realises there's no energy available in the stomach, it will change tactics and take the required energy from your *fat stores* instead. That's right, your body will automatically use your *body fat* as energy, burning it away without you having to do *any extra work*. Obviously, the actual

process is a bit more in-depth than that, but I don't want to complicate things with a load of scientific mumbo jumbo right now.

Note: There's a whole chapter on "The science behind fasting" further along in the book for you to read if you're the sort of person who needs to know exactly why something works. But for now, I'm just going to assume that you're not a scientifically-minded person, or that the "basics" will suffice. Also, I'm not going to force you to read "boring" scientific stuff if you don't want to. I'm nice like that, lol.

So, now you know; you can lose that nasty, unwanted body fat by simply changing your eating schedule. Sounds too easy, doesn't it? Well it is! It absolutely, positively *is* that easy to lose excess fat, to become leaner and healthier whilst still enjoying nice-tasting (or "unhealthy") foods. This is one of the most simple and effective methods that you will find to get rid of that unwanted body fat whilst, as an added bonus, retaining all of the good bodyweight (bone, muscle, organs) and turning your body into a naturally efficient, lean, mean, fat-burning machine!

The reason so many people easily succeed at becoming leaner by using an intermittent fasting plan, is because there are very few "behavioural" changes required to make these huge physical results happen. You don't have to give up the things that you like (tasty food), you don't have to do things that you don't like (running, eating salad for every meal, etc.), and calorie-counting? (*shudder*) I don't think so! Nope, all you have to do is make a tiny tweak to your eating schedule and watch the fat melt away. Easy-peasy!

This process is so simple that you'll definitely be able to do it, yet it's so effective that you'll hardly believe your eyes when you see the results! You'll feel good and you'll look great! You may even end up looking so amazing that you'll drown in a sea of people wanting to sex you up...

Disclaimer – I cannot actually guarantee that you'll literally drown in an ocean of sexy-time, but the likelihood of this is probably dramatically increased if you lose fat and become more sexually-confident.

So why 'hypno' fasting?
Fasting itself is great, it works really well. So, if you skipped the hypnosis portion of this book, and only focused on the fasting part, you'd still lose weight, that's a given. However, our minds can have a massive effect on many things, including both our psychology (mood, willpower, mindset, etc.) and also our physiology (body processes). Harnessing the power of your mind in order to make your fat-loss process easier and more effective is a no-brainer... or, a brainer, I guess... but I'll talk more about that in the "Programming Your Mind for Success" section later on in the book, after you learn how to fast.

What you *need* to do…
If, after reading this brief introductory chapter, you've made up your mind that you're definitely ready to get rid of your excess fat, and that you're going to give this awesome plan a go (which you probably are, because you're still reading), then all I ask is that you'll follow these 2 ridiculously simple rules:

RULE 1:
Start doing this shit ASAP

Don't think about "when it would be best to start…"
The best time is now! Don't waste your *precious* time thinking about it… Just do it. Seriously, the time is now… we'll be dead soon.

Don't think about "what social engagements might coincide with it…"
Unless you're a hermit (the person, not the crab), then there are *always* going to be social engagements, so suck it up and get on with it.

Don't say "I'll start next Monday…"
Starting "next Monday" is like waiting for the New Year to make a resolution; it's stupid, because you're only cheating yourself out of more time in your new, leaner, healthier body!

So, start as soon as you possibly can, because why wouldn't you? You want to change, don't you? If you answered no, then put this book down and go grab yourself a pie (or ten) and come back when you're ready to accept that *you* are responsible for making changes happen in your life, not me, not this book, not your partner, your doctor, your life coach or your great aunt Maud. YOU are responsible! So, if you can start tomorrow, start tomorrow. If you can't start tomorrow, ask yourself, honestly, why the hell not? Are you going to be busy competing in a 24-hour eating contest? I highly doubt it (but, if so, good luck). #EatAllTheThings

Start now, today, and quit making BS excuses for yourself. This fasting program is not complicated, the only reason it won't work is if you don't actually do it…

So just…
Fucking…
Do it!

(…see what I mean about that push in the right direction? …and the swearing? I wasn't joking, lol.)

After you follow rule 1 and you've actually started on your intermittent fasting plan, you're going to want to follow rule 2 for maximum effectiveness…

RULE 2:
You need to be consistent (ish)

Now, in a lot of diets consistency can be a really big problem. Often, it can be a big enough problem to completely screw up the diet, causing the dieter to quit, for example; someone on a low-carb diet completely surrendering to their cravings and demolishing a whole double chocolate cheesecake with a side order of guilt...

There's often that "fuck it" moment at some point during a typical diet, which happens due to being forced to do too much of something that you don't really want to do, and that's when the old-fashioned "diet" completely falls apart. With the plans in this book however, you get a lot more freedom. So long as you stick to your IF plan *most* of the time, the odd "fuck it" won't make a significant difference because, unlike a diet, it's easy to go back to your fasting plan.

Unlike a diet, you won't feel such a huge pang of guilt if you accidentally (or purposefully) "fuck it" once every few weeks. If you go on a week-long eating binge however, don't expect the results to be so forgiving. I'll give you some more specific examples when we go over the full plans later on in the book, but just remember; you get out what you put in. If you're shitty at sticking to the plan, your results are going to be shitty, you're going to look shitty and that's going to make you feel shitty... and that would be pretty darn shitty, right? #IMayHaveTourettes

So, I've told you that these plans are easy, and they are, but you're still going to have to use a *little bit* of willpower, at least initially. As with all changes in habit, the first few days may *seem* a little tough, the reason for this is quite simple; it's something that you're not used to doing. In reality, these plans are probably very different from the eating plan that you've been force-fed (pun intended) by modern society to accept as "normal" for most of your life (3 square meals a day, anyone?), and because you have no evidence from your past experiences to tell you whether this "new thing" is a good idea (and more importantly whether it will reward you in a way that you would like), your sneaky, sneaky mind may try to convince you to give up before you've even begun. Yes, your mind might *try* to trick you back into your "normal" eating habits...

But wait! Don't reprimand your brain just yet, because I have good news for you; this "tough part" isn't *actually* that tough at all! For instance, it's nowhere near as tough as a calorie-restriction diet or 2-hours-a-day on the treadmill, that's for sure! Transitioning to this plan is a piece of cake in comparison. The second piece of ~~cake~~ good news is that the "(not so) tough part" is only temporary! When I personally began to use intermittent fasting, it only took me about 3 days to really get into the swing of it!

Those sexy science-nerds tell us that a new habit can be fully formed in *around* 21 days, so whether it's just 3 days or 3 short weeks into your new eating plan, you might find that it will already have started to become almost second nature to you. Also, when you get to the 3-week point, you will probably have already noticed a reduction of your body fat, which will give you all the more motivation to continue to enjoy this awesome, easy new way of eating normal food and burning fat like a boss!

So, if you choose to follow the 2 rules I just mentioned, then successfully losing fat using this process is easy. There are, however, a couple of other things that you could *choose to do*, to help speed up the fat-loss process quite dramatically…

What you don't "*need*" to do…
You don't *need* to give up eating junk food, and you don't *need* to eat healthy meals, but *if* you are able to ditch the Mc-Pizza-Fried-Taco-King… *If* you can reduce your binge-drinking a little and drink more water instead… *If* you can cut out snacking on sticks of butter and bags of sugar in between meals… These small dietary modifications will help your fat-burning machine (body) to become much more efficient at burning fat (and the fat-burning process will happen a lot faster too), but like I said, it's optional. You

don't *need* to eat healthier food to lose weight when fasting, but if you decide that you'd like to help the process along and burn fat more efficiently, there's a whole chapter near the end of the book called "How to Eat Healthier" that will point you in the right direction.

You definitely don't *need* to exercise for this plan to work, but again, if you want faster results and if you really want to feel fit and *look good naked*, then it's recommended that you do some kind of cardio and resistance/weight training alongside your fasting plan. Now, I'm not suggesting that you need to make yourself look like an 80's Arnold Schwarzenegger (unless you constantly feel an inexplicable need to GET TO A CHOPPA), but it is a scientific fact that if you have more muscle, the fat will drop off of you faster, because muscle naturally burns more calories than fat, *so more muscle = good*.

If weight training ain't for you (and you should totally try it before you decide), then cardio might be more up your street... Again, you can tell me to cram it where the sun doesn't shine, but from my own personal experience, this stuff works (the exercise, not the butt-cramming), and though some of them may deny it, members of the opposite sex (or the same sex, if you'd prefer ...or both if you're greedy) are programmed to appreciate fit physical specimens, so if that's not motivation then I don't know what is!

If you would like to learn more about what sort of exercises will or won't help you to reach your body-goals, then check out the "How to Exercise" section at the back of the book. It has details on both weight training and dirty, dirty cardio, so you can choose whichever you like. Or, alternatively, you can choose to tear that section out, rip it up into tiny little pieces, set it on fire and go and have a little sit down.

Like I said before, this shit is all up to you.

You da boss.

Why Most "Diets" Suck

I'm going to lump *all diets* into one big group here, because whether calorie counting, high protein, low carb, high fat, Atkins, Slimming World, Cambridge, Paleo, South Beach, juice only, banana-only (seriously), or anything else, fundamentally; diets is diets. It doesn't really matter which type of diet you choose, because no matter the type, there are often similar challenges and outcomes during and after dieting. Diets *can* work, I'm not saying they don't, what I'm saying is that for many people they only tend to work on a temporary basis. It's often hard to stick to a diet long-term (especially if it's low-calories or low-carb based), and if you go off your diet for even a day or two, you almost-immediately fuck up all your hard-earned progress... What a waste of time, effort and sanity!

With the IF process however, you *do* have a long-term solution. Yes, you *are* putting stress on your body (like with many of the other diets), but it's only a relatively small amount of stress. Once you've done the fasting bit, you can then replenish your energy stores (and your emotional health) by eating whatever type of food your body needs, wants, craves, and loves, rather than just gobbling 30 more bananas like a brain-damaged chimpanzee. Also, if you take a couple of days off, it isn't such a big deal. You will notice that, of the 3 techniques suggested in this book, only 1 of them is an "every day" kinda deal. If you use the "Weekender Plan" for instance, you will only be fasting for around 8 days per month! Sounds good right? (We'll come to the plans shortly).

Some diets tell us to "eat less and exercise more", but on what planet does that advice make sense (unless your aim is to completely screw yourself over)? If you are (properly) engaging in exercise, you are automatically going to be burning a LOT more calories than the average couch potato. To allow your muscles to recover, and to actually give your body a fighting chance, you would in fact need to add *extra* fuel to compensate for that exercise, so "eating less" is not a smart idea. Eating less than your body requires whilst engaging in exercise means your muscles will deplete and your immune system will probably quit on you too, due to too much stress! You don't see world-class powerlifters and bodybuilders on those 600-calorie-a-day liquid shake diets, do you? (no). In fact, some of those guys eat upwards of 10,000 calories a day (which is 4x the amount of the average human male's recommended daily intake). #SignMeUp

Another thing that sucks about normal diets, is that they often cause you to lose "weight" as opposed to the thing you actually want to do, which is lose "fat". You don't want to lose muscle, in fact it's beneficial for you to have more muscle (as mentioned before). To build muscle your body needs excess calories (and a pretty high protein intake too), so, if you're eating

600 calories per day, not only will you *not* be able to build muscle, your body will actually be cannibalizing the muscle that you already have (for energy). From the perspective of someone who might want a bit of extra muscle to help aid fat-loss... that sucks.

With intermittent fasting, you have the option to exercise (*if you want to),* and once you're done you can then fuel your body with as much food as it needs. So rather than "eat less and exercise more", an intermittent fasting mantra would be more like "eat less OFTEN and exercise when you want to". Even if you *don't* plan on exercising, long-term, daily calorific restriction is still a completely stupid idea! If a diet is telling you to eat less than around 50% of your recommended daily calorie intake, day-in, day-out, alarm bells should be ringing. It's called a *recommended* calorie intake for a reason you know!

FYI, if you didn't know; the "average male" (whatever that is) should be eating around 2,500 calories per day, and it's around 2,000 calories per day for (average) females. If you dramatically cut your calories for any extended period of time, your body will realise this and it will automatically increase your appetite to try and remedy the problem (because your body is smarter than whoever came up with that stupid diet).

My own personal calorie intake (at the time of writing) is around 3,000-3,500 calories per day, because I lift weights 2-3 times a week and I want to build muscle. Staying relatively lean whilst eating pretty much whatever I want is a good result. Most people (on standard diets) would have to carefully calculate their macronutrients (protein, fat & carbohydrate) ratio to attain such a goal. Luckily for us, with intermittent fasting you don't have to do that!

Note: There's nothing stopping you from calculating your "macros" alongside these IF plans. If you're happy to calculate your meal/calorie/macronutrient amounts, this can potentially help you to achieve results faster – but it's definitely not for everyone!

So, diets on the whole are a pretty dull and soul-destroying pastime. You're punished for eating things you like, and what about the rewards for doing the terribly boring, uncomfortable stuff you don't like? Well, they usually take ages to come about and are fragile and fuck-upable. You are given limited food choices, you can end up with nutritional deficiencies by not being allowed to eat certain types of food, and some of these diets are downright embarrassing;

"Sorry, I can't have a piece of that cake you made especially for my birthday, because I'm on a diet."

"No, I can't even have just one drink with you guys, because I've given up alcohol forever! Urgh!"

"I'd love to have a slice of pizza, but my diet doesn't allow foods with carbs, and I kinda want to die…"

Screw that! You shouldn't have to explain your eating habits, you shouldn't need to have your life limited by diets, and you *definitely* shouldn't have to stop having fun because of them!

Take a moment and compare everything that you know about diets, all of the sacrifices, the struggles, the inner turmoil, in comparison to intermittent fasting, where you simply change your meal timing or reduce your calories *intermittently*, whilst continuing to eat the stuff that you actually like… Well that seems a lot more agreeable, doesn't it?!

All in all, I think we can agree that standard diets are not the ideal choice for you to achieve long-term success, and by getting rid of all the complications of dieting, ditching all the restrictions and turning your back on all of the other tedious, needlessly uncomfortable shit, you are much more likely to succeed. **Hypno-Fasting** is much more fun and much easier on you as a human being! Also, by fasting and having more variety in what you eat, this will actually promote better health and you'll be happier too (obviously). #DontWorryBeHappy

Positive Benefits and Possible "Side Effects"

So, as with *most* things in life, there are potential negative aspects as well as positive ones, and it is our duty (to ourselves) to weigh up the pros and cons and figure out whether it's beneficial for us to do something or to choose an alternative that might work better for us as individuals. In the case of intermittent fasting, the list of positive effects *enormously* outweighs the possible "side effects", and in my experience, *most* people won't suffer any side effects, but it's a good idea to have all of the information at hand so that *you* can make your own informed decision – don't just take my word for it, feel free to do some research! So, let's start with the positive effects of intermittent fasting:

Fast, effective fat-loss
Well, the #1 positive effect of this technique (and probably the reason that you picked up this book) is obviously the fast, effective fat-loss potential (#CaptainObvious). It is easily possible to lose up to 2lb of excess fat per week – this number is entirely subjective to the individual in question, as we all naturally burn fat at different rates due to our different body types, metabolisms, activity levels, etc. Also, food & exercise choices play a substantial part in the rate at which fat will be burnt. Still, even with that in mind, intermittent fasting (when used

properly) will melt the fat right off, and above all; it's easy (...I think I've drummed that point in enough though, so we'll move on).

Long-term low-body-fat maintenance solution
The 3 plans in this book are easy to maintain over long periods of time or even indefinitely, because this way of eating is completely natural. So not only are you *not* starving yourself of things that you want/need, you're probably going to become even healthier than before you used this plan. I know of a great many people who use the IF eating model and have done so for years and years whilst maintaining a lean, healthy physique and feeling fantastic. This IF plan does not take a toll on the body in the same way as a calorie-restrictive diet would. You don't feel groggy and crappy. In fact, during the "fasting" period, a lot of people experience even higher energy levels and become more focused than normal – strange but true!

A flexible approach
You have 3 different choices/plans that are easy to tailor around any type of lifestyle. You can choose from the following:

The Full-Timer Plan
(Highly Recommended)
Eat for 8 hours, fast for 16, repeat every day.

The 50% Plan
Eat "normally" for 1 day, eat 500-600 calories the next, alternate continuously.

The Weekender Plan
Eat "normally" for 5 days, eat 500-600 calories for 2 days, repeat.

I'll go into greater detail about those shortly, but I thought I'd show you the options now to give you a rough idea of what to expect, and to demonstrate that there are 3 *very different* eating plans for you to pick from. There's no "one-size-fits-all" plan, because we're not all the same size (if we were, I wouldn't be writing this book).

Alongside the 3 different eating plans, there is even more flexibility, because unlike dieting, you are able to easily "pick up and put down" your fasting plan as-and-when you need to. With standard dieting, if you go on holiday for a week and pig out on everything on offer (because, fuck it, it's a holiday, right?), coming home and giving up treats again is going to SUCK! But coming home and eating exactly the same stuff as normal, just at different times? Well, that ain't nothin' but plain sailin', baby!

I personally like to take a break over the "festive period" because I like to eat Xmas food with the family and then get drunk (woo hoo!), but then as soon as Xmas is over, you can get straight back on it for the next year (or most of it). This Xmas-break isn't something I "recommend", but I mention it to let you know that these plans are well within the realms of possibility for almost anyone, and they're easily modifiable to suit your own goals, lifestyle and personal commitments.

Note: Just know that putting some excess body fat back on during the winter doesn't (psychologically) feel great after being leaner for the rest of the year! lol

Easy and simple to do
Why would anyone choose a complicated "diet" that stresses them out? Constantly working out how many calories are in every morsel of food... Having to read the tiny "calorie contents" table on the back of everything you buy at the supermarket... That's just the tip of the iceberg. Some people can tolerate that type of diet, some people even thrive within such a confined and structured plan, but I hate it, and I guess you do too, so let's keep it simple!

If you use the first IF plan that I recommend, you'll get 8 hours a day to eat – that basically equates to two meals (for example: lunch @ 12noon & evening meal @ 7.30pm), so you're automatically making your life simpler by cutting out one meal. You're cutting out 33% of the stress of "what should I eat?" and you're cutting out 33% of the stress of food preparation, cooking, eating and washing the dishes, all of which takes valuable time out of your day. You're cutting your food bill down too, not only because you're "skipping" a meal, but also because…

You don't get as hungry
Sounds counter-intuitive, doesn't it? You'd think that eating 2 meals instead of 3 would cause an increase in hunger, but it doesn't, in fact it does the absolute frigging opposite! Once you are attuned to the way that your body reacts to food (by fasting), you'll soon realise that "hunger" is often not hunger at all, but just boredom! Too many people are getting fat because they're bored senseless and just eating for the sake of boredom! The first couple of days into fasting, you might *think* you're hungry, but you'll drink a glass of water and realise that you're not actually hungry at all. Eventually, you'll naturally realise when you're hungry and when you're not, and honestly, that old hunger thing won't bother you half as much as it might at the moment.

Sometimes during my daily fast, it gets to my usual eating-time (around 1pm) and I find that I'm not even remotely hungry. When this happens I do something miraculous, and something that the old, 3-meal-a-day me would never have done, I simply DON'T EAT! This is some revolutionary shit right here, eh? If your body doesn't actually require food, your newly attuned mind won't make you think you're hungry, so you won't even want to eat. You will then have much more time on your hands, which you can use to do something *productive*, instead of wasting time eating for no good reason!

You can build/retain muscle
I already mentioned it, but if you go to the gym (or if you want to start), then the plans in this book are completely suitable to use alongside a resistance training program. You're gonna get enough calories to build and retain muscle, whilst ensuring excess body fat drops/remains low, and you can time your fasting plan around your workouts for maximum effectiveness!

You really can build a lot of muscle whilst using this technique – I've personally gained around 45lb (20kg) of muscle whilst using the "Full-Timer Plan". You're probably not going to get hugely muscular (i.e. the size of the Incredible Hulk) while using these plans, but you are definitely able to become impressively muscular if you want to (well, assuming you put some effort into it).

Let's have a bunch of health-benefits too
Calorie restriction is a way of causing the body to extend its natural life-span (i.e. when you eat less than your daily recommended amount of calories, your body will slow down its own biological ageing processes). Long-term calorie restriction, however, is not something that we want to do because it is unpleasant, and if you do it long-term, those positive benefits will soon be outweighed by the negatives.

Luckily, similar positive results are achievable through intermittent fasting. A recent study (2017) at Harvard showed that intermittent fasting might lead to prolonged lifespans too ...which is nice! (Google "Fasting Harvard lifespan" if you want to read it.)

Various studies have also suggested that intermittent fasting has many health benefits, such as; improved insulin sensitivity, improved resistance to infections/ diseases, improved immune system, reduced risk of arthritis, reduced inflammation, and even a reduction in menopausal issues such as hot-flushes (sorry guys, there's no cure for mid-life-crisis symptoms... unless you count getting a ripped 6-pack, of course). There has also been extensive research into the link between fasting and diseases, which has suggested that intermittent fasting noticeably reduces the risk of cardiovascular (heart) disease, diabetes, and has even been shown to reduce the risk of cancer too.

Note: I'm not saying this eating plan will cure cancer, give you a natural heart-transplant or raise the dead 'n' shit. However, it definitely makes a lot of people (myself included) feel healthier, so hopefully this plan will help you to feel healthier and live longer too – no promises though. #Soz

So those are some of the positive effects of fasting, now let's cover the possibility of side effects. I do not know of any scientific studies that have taken place to prove/disprove the following possible side effects, so all of the points I have included are "anecdotal", meaning people have said that these things happened, but there's no *real* way to know whether they were related to intermittent fasting, or whether they were caused by something else. This is because the reports were all personal-circumstances and didn't take into account any other activities that they might have been engaging in at the time.

Possible negative effects:
- Irritability/anxiety
- Difficulty sleeping/too much energy
- Tiredness/faintness/reduced energy
- Bad breath (common with low-carb diets)
- Dehydration (drink more water, genius)
- Raised/lowered blood-pressure (weight loss in general can alter blood pressure)
- Reduced body temperature (less fat = less insulation)

Note: Again, just to remind you; intermittent fasting is not recommended for pregnant women (also women who are breastfeeding). There have been no studies (to my knowledge) including participants of extreme ages (i.e. younger than 18 and older than 65), so in these cases be aware that risk of negative consequences could possibly be increased...maybe?

So, there you have it. There are *possible* side effects (both positive and negative) and it's up to you to figure out if this plan is right for you. You can believe what I say (which is based on *my* personal experience, and research), or if you want to learn more, you can go and do some research of your own. There's plenty out there to choose from, but my advice to you (and the way that I initially approached fasting) is that a little research is good, but you're never going to know what works for *you* until you try it for yourself. You can read a hundred shitty reviews of a movie, then watch the movie yourself and absolutely love it. You know why? Because sometimes other people are just plain wrong! Sometimes you have to bite the bullet and make your own decisions. Carve your own path to a better life by doing what works for you, and if you try something new and it sucks, well at least you tried and you aren't just blindly going along with what other people tell you to do. Often, though, you'll find that many of these new experiences turn out to be some of the best things you'll ever do, and you may even wonder why you didn't start sooner!

Positive Effects Recap:
- Fast, effective fat-loss
- Long-term low body fat maintenance solution
- Flexible & easy to maintain
- Easy to understand & easy to do
- Reduced feeling of hunger
- Great for building/maintaining muscle mass
- Possible additional health-benefits

The Science Behind Fasting

OK, so you've got to this point and you're still reading. Well done! Now, here comes the science behind the plans. You don't *need* to know this stuff for these plans to work, so if you don't want to read this section, no pressure! Do keep in mind, however, that this section will still be written in the same way as the rest of the book, because learning about science doesn't have to be dull! So, let's continue...

Supposedly, the "modern version" of intermittent fasting (that we know) was "discovered" by accident when some crazy scientific bastards (Carlson & Hoelzel) were attempting to increase the life-span of rats. When subjected to intermittent fasting tests, these rats were observed to have lower body fat, less hunger, a longer life and a reduced risk of diseases and diabetes...

There have, however, been many non-scientific occurrences of fasting throughout various different cultures and religions in the past, the most notable of which being the Islamic holy month of Ramadan. The Ramadan fast has supposedly been happening all over the world for over 1,400 years. Participants fast from the moment they wake up, all the way through to sunset, and then continue to eat what they'd normally eat (though Muslims *also* abstain from sexual relations and profanity during their Ramadan fasting, but *you* don't have to do that! lol). So, as well as a method of fat-loss and "physical cleansing", some think of fasting as a "spiritual experience" too.

OK, that's not science, that's more like history...

Science, bitch!
So, what's the difference between fasting and being fed-up (i.e. always eating)? If you're eating 3 meals a day (and probably snacking too) your body is constantly in a fed-up state. After eating food, it generally takes between 3-5 hours for that food to be digested. While your body is actively digesting all the food that you crammed into it, fat burning is pretty much out of the question, this is due to the fact that your insulin levels are probably high, and insulin's job is to regulate energy stores. The more sensitive you are to insulin, the more efficiently your body will use your food. So, if there's food in your body, your body is going to use that for fuel, rather than focusing on your fat stores. Makes sense, right?

After the food is completely digested and absorbed, you are then into the "post-absorptive state" (which simply means "after your food is absorbed" ...who'd have guessed?), so although the digestion process is over in 3-5 hours, the actual fast doesn't get into full-swing until around 12 hours after your last meal. How often, during modern day-to-day life do we have a period of 12 consecutive hours with no food/drink? Not very often at all (for most people), hence most people who eat "normally" have probably *never* experienced the benefits of fasting.

So, around 12 hours (give or take) after your last meal, your body goes into fast-mode. During this fast state, your body doesn't have additional glucose in your blood or glycogen in your liver/muscles to use as fuel, so instead it will begin to utilise the excess fat stored within your body. This is why, once in the fast state, it becomes easier for your body to burn fat. Whoop whoop!

Note: This is also why exercising whilst fasted is said to be more effective at burning fat than "regular exercise", because if you don't have a pre-workout meal, more fat will have to be used to fuel that crazy shit you're doing. Also, for the muscle-builders amongst you, fasting naturally increases secretion of growth hormones, leading to better muscular gains... #TheMoreYouKnow

Being in a fast state also naturally improves your insulin sensitivity, thereby causing your body to more effectively use the food that you put into it after "breaking fast" (...yes, that's why it's called "breakfast"). Also, I mentioned glycogen; your body *can* use this as fuel, but it is naturally depleted after a good night's sleep (and even more so after a fast), which again means that your body is going to skip that choice and go straight for the fat stores! Bonus!

Go eat yourself!
There is another process caused by intermittent fasting, known as "autophagy" (the literal translation meaning "self-eating"). This is a process whereby cells create a package of enzymes (called Lysosomes) that are used to find unwanted/diseased cells in the body and destroy them. Why? Because the lack of food during a fast means the body has to find alternative fuel sources from within itself, and one of the most obvious things that the body can do without is unhealthy cells! Unfortunately for most people, the older we get, the more the autophagy process is naturally reduced, and by not-fasting (i.e. eating "normally") it is reduced even more, making it much easier for us to get sick and/or dead. So, by fasting, we naturally (and safely) increase the autophagy process and as a result, increase our body's ability to "self-cleanse", meaning that whilst fasting your body is going to be one happy camper!

A lot of "diets" can end up with you becoming run-down and even unhealthier than when you began, but fasting does exactly the opposite, helping you to lose unwanted fat whilst also becoming healthier. An amazing combination. Now if only we can figure out how it can make us rich and get us laid too. Oh, talking of sex...

Men vs. Women
Intermittent fasting affects men and women slightly differently, and IF is (generally) slightly more

beneficial for men as a rule, but don't assume that it won't work for women, because it has and does! You've got to keep in mind, that we humans are all very different from one another, and what works well for some does not work so well for others. It has been said that while men experience an improvement in insulin sensitivity whilst fasting, women do not (or experience less). There has also been evidence of a positive effect on male blood lipids (fats) that was not found in female results.

Men and women are quite different (even though some guys *have* managed to grow their own boobs), so we can't assume that making the same dietary changes will cause the same results across the board. Look at bodybuilders, for instance; the male body is naturally able to achieve enormous sizes, while the female form is not as well adapted for this, and will usually, be less naturally muscular – that's why *big* female body builders that use a ton of steroids look so... uh... unique. #TactfulAsFuck

Again, there are always exceptions to the rule, as with most things, but the exception is *not the rule*. So, just because a very small number of women may have gotten less results from fasting, this doesn't mean that many *other women* can't get massive benefits from it ...and the best way to get those benefits is to go out and do it!

...that old chestnut again. Heh.

Other sciency stuff…
Many people believe that they are "cursed" with
poor genetics, that they are naturally inclined to be
obese, and that woe-unto-me, there is nothing that
can be done! Might as well grab a family sized bucket
of fried greasy crap and chow down, eh?! Well
actually, no! "Genetics" is no longer a valid excuse…

Epigenetics (the study of cellular and physiological
trait variations that are *not caused* by changes in the
DNA sequence) have shown that the human
mind/body is able to overcome "genetics" by
creating new habits (such as an intermittent fasting
plan). So just because your entire family are fat and
lazy, doesn't mean you have to be. How you choose
to live, how you act and react during your day-to-day
life is much more important than "what you've
inherited". So, if you've ever used "genetics" as an
excuse, I suggest you quit whining like a stubborn
child and do something about it! #MicrophoneDrop

Intermittent fasting makes you smarter
No, I'm not even joking. The fasting process
increases "BDNF" (Brain-derived neurotrophic
factor), a protein which increases brain growth.
Increasing BDNF allows for better "connections"
within your mind/body that create the potential for
you to become more intelligent. Why does this
happen? Well, if you were a brain, and you were
going to die because the body you were in wasn't
smart enough to find food, wouldn't you want to

make the body a bit smarter so that it could find something to eat? I know I would!

Modern eating habits make us stupider, because we don't need to "hunt" for our food, we don't need to scavenge or forage for sustenance. Nope, all you need to do is remember to grab your wallet (or even just your phone) before you venture out into the vast and terrifying human wasteland known as "grocery shopping"! So, the very least you can do is use fasting to trick your brain into thinking that you're hunting, when in fact you're probably just watching funny cat videos online and scratching yourself whilst some poor soul on a pizza delivery bike tries to find your lazy ass in 30 minutes or less (otherwise it's FREE)!

Before microwave dinners, before World Wars, before religion, and before organised language, our ancient ancestors were often only able to eat "intermittently" due to the fact that there were no McMammoth burgers, 500-calorie beverages, or refrigerators full of processed, hydrogenous fluorescent crap that doesn't naturally exist (and barely manages to pass itself off as "food" at all)! Those ancient hunter-gatherers were not blessed/ cursed with any of that crap. Our Neolithic ancestors needed to function at optimum level (physically as well as mentally) during periods without food, otherwise they'd go hungry and starve to death. Because of this inherent need to sustain ourselves,

our ancient bodies adapted and evolved to work optimally whilst (unwittingly) utilising intermittent fasting. So, let's carry the torch for our half-man/half-ape ancestors, with intermittent fasting. I mean, those guys were strong, shredded and beat the shit out of Sabre-Toothed Tigers... what more could you want from a role model? Oh, they didn't have a Twitter account? Boo bloody hoo!
#HashtagsAreOverratedAnyway #IronicHashtag #AmITrendingYet?

How to Fast

There are many different schools of thought on the subject of fasting, and there are too many people trying to peddle their own "new" and "ground-breaking" fasting plans, when in fact the big 3 (covered in this book) are the most effective. These 3 plans are tried-and-tested, and they actually work. They are proven by science (like, scientifically and everything), so why try and change something that already works great? (...well, probably because they want to make some money, that's why.) Don't listen to the snake-oil salesmen, scammers, and the people who're trying to re-invent the wheel, when you can go straight to the source!

The 3 plans that I have set out in this book are the very best fasting solutions available to you, the discriminating reader. All *good* fasting books will be promoting one (or more) of these 3 plans, and although these *are* the very same plans that have been detailed and used extensively by fasting enthusiasts across the globe for years, I've re-named them because, well, it's my book, so I do what I want. #RebelRebel

Here are your 3 awesome options:

- The Full-Timer Plan
- The 50% Plan
- The Weekender Plan

Let's go over the 3 plans in a little more detail – I suggest that you read through *all 3 plans* (even if you've already decided which one you're going to do before you've read them), because they each contain awesome nuggets of information that can be used regardless of the plan that you choose...

The Full-Timer Plan (Recommended)

Sometimes known as: 8 Hour / 16:8
Brief summary: Eat for 8 hours, fast for 16, repeat every day.

The Full-Timer Plan is probably the best choice for a consistent, effective intermittent fasting solution. The idea is that you set yourself a daily "eating window" and keep it consistent, day-in, day-out. This plan can easily be tailored to suit most lifestyles (and jobs). This is my absolute favourite fasting plan, and it's the one that I personally use.

How to do the Full-Timer Plan
Firstly, you'll need to figure out if this is the right plan for you. Do you have a fairly regular schedule, or are you able to make time to fit your dietary arrangements around your life? Yes? If so, this plan should be your go-to choice. Once you've done the maths and figured out if this plan will work for you (it does for most people), you'll then need to decide exactly when your daily 8-hour eating window should take place. The most popular choice is frequently 12noon until 8pm or thereabouts, some people go 11am-7pm or 1pm-9pm, but it all depends on you! Make the plan fit your life, not the other way around.

*Note: If you are a **female**, it's suggested that you have a slightly longer eating window of around 10 hours, meaning a 14 hour fast instead of 16 hours.*

Again, this is just suggested, so feel free to ignore this suggestion, but many women tend to find that 14:10 (or even 15:9) timing works a little better with the female body. #NotSexismJustFacts

If you prefer to eat in the mornings to fuel your day, and you don't frequently eat in the evening anyway, then it might be more sensible to start eating at breakfast time and go through to the afternoon (i.e. a 7am-3pm eating window) and then fast. But if you, like me, frequently find yourself getting hungry in the evening, then fasting *all evening* is not a very sensible option. So, skipping breakfast (and that's all it really is; skipping breakfast) and eating in the afternoon/evening is gonna be the more sensible choice for you.

I'm sure you've already got an idea of when your preferred eating window is most likely to be, now it's just a case of getting on with it. The "meal frequency" that most people adopt during their 8 hours is to have just two meals, one at the start (let's say 1pm for example) and then the second meal at around a half hour before you intend to begin fasting again (so around 8:30pm in this example), this gives you a comfortable 30 minutes in which to eat your second meal. Also, worth mentioning is that it's common practice to cut out snacking and "grazing" when you're using a fasting plan. Initially this is done on purpose, because obviously the less calories you're eating, the more fat you'll be burning, but also because once you get "into the swing" of fasting, you genuinely find that eating (snacking specifically) takes a back-seat in your life. This means you find yourself thinking less about food, and then you naturally end up snacking less anyway. Which is great news if you want to lose some fat!

So that's the "feeding" part, what about the "fasting" part...
The Full-Timer Plan is the only plan in the book that utilises a proper fast (as you will see when you read the other two plans). You will be doing what's known as a "water fast", which means during your fasting period, you'll eat absolutely no food, and you should only drink water. Well, actually you can have tea and coffee too, but you'll have to ditch the milk and sugar, because they contain calories (in case you didn't know). Black tea/coffee is a great option, because it helps you to feel full, and like you've had something more substantial than water (also, a bit of caffeine is useful in aiding fat-loss too). If you don't like hot drinks, you can even chug a *diet (0 calorie)* soda (if you like that fizzy shit, and don't care whether you have any teeth left in 10 years).

Just remember, you are aiming for a calorie intake of 0 (that's ZERO CALORIES) during the fasting period, and it surprises me just how often people overlook the fact that drinks contain calories. For example:

Large Mc Coke = 280 calories
(Over 10% of your daily calories)

Large Orange Juice = 280 calories
(What? But it's made of fruit! Yup, fruit has calories)

Large Mocha Coffee = 450 calories
(Almost, a QUARTER of your daily calories)

Black Tea/Coffee = 0 Calories
(But only if you don't put milk and sugar in it)

Water = 0 calories
(Get the point?)

You may well be drinking more liquids than normal whilst fasting, so do keep in mind that you might have to use the bathroom more frequently (this isn't a bad thing, because you're actually "flushing" a load of crap out of your body, but it's not always convenient to be pissing like a racehorse all day long).

So, why specifically 16:8 hours?
You do not have to stick rigidly to the 16:8 model. You don't need to sit there with a stopwatch, making sure you get it dead-on every day. 16 hours is your suggested minimum fasting duration (for men). Fasting for less than your 16 hours is pretty much a waste of time, because as mentioned previously, the benefits of fasting only *fully* begin after around 12

hours of not eating. So, with a 16 hour fast, you are getting 4 solid hours of full fasting benefits, fast for any less time, and your results can suffer quite dramatically. You can, however, go the other way and have a slightly longer fast... Obviously, the longer the fast, the faster the results (someone doing 20:4 fasting will lose weight faster than someone doing 16:8), some crazy bastards will even have just one *large* meal a day, and fast for the rest of the time!

I find fasting for over 20 hours to be a bit much, but sometimes it can be good to mix it up... You can do 16:8 as standard, and sometimes stick a 17-20 hour fast in there, but only if you want to. The 16:8 timing is designed to make it easy and comfortable, so that you are able to eat with your friends/family, allowing you to have a seemingly "normal" life, whilst benefitting from a sensible, sustainable IF plan.

Note: Anything over 24 hours, and you're getting into "long-fasting" territory, which will be covered at the end of this chapter – please read that section, because it is very important.

"16 hours with no food seems like a long time!"
Ordinarily, 16 hours with no food might seem like a bit of a chore, but you've got to remember that you're probably going to be fast asleep (no pun intended) during your fast, so depending on how much sleep you get, you'll probably only be fasting for a relatively short amount of time:

5 hours sleep = 11 hour fast
6 hours sleep = 10 hour fast
7 hours sleep = 9 hour fast
8 hours sleep = 8 hour fast
9 hours sleep = 7 hour fast

Honestly, a 16 hour fast is easy. The first couple of days may seem like you had to put in a little bit of effort to achieve your goal, but soon it becomes almost second nature, to the point where you'll barely even think about it at all, and when you realise that, it will feel pretty damn good!

The "Fuck It" Moment
Most people are fallible (i.e. we make mistakes), even those "perfect" people who must literally just be out there to try and make us look bad in comparison, yes, they fuck up too. Everyone fucks up, and there's no way around that. There *will* be times when you won't be able to stick to the plan, all I am going to ask you to do, Is do your best. If you have to go to a wedding and have a wedding-breakfast at 8am with the bride/groom, but you're meant to be fasting until 1pm... Fuck it! The wedding is more important than 1 day of fasting.

The point is, you have a life! The great thing about IF is that it's super easy to work around life ...most of the time. Sometimes the shit will hit the fan, but so long as you're not having a "fuck it" moment every day or two, then you're gonna make progress.

As well as sticking to the plan *as much as you can,* you also need to ensure that your priorities are right, and that you have damage control in place. So, if you *must* eat outside your eating window, you can always choose a healthier option, instead of the greasy bacon, sausage and lard sandwich or the 2lb triple-bypass-cheeseburger. Otherwise, you could always make up for the "fuck it" moment by having a slightly longer fast the next day, or eating slightly less than normal during your next eating window…

You've got to remember, if you fuck it all the time, the only thing you're truly fucking is yourself.

Please don't fuck yourself…

…especially not in public.

"The Full-Timer Plan" – Key Points:

- Fast for at least 16 hours per 24-hour period (or 14-16 hours for females)
- No food/calorific drinks during the fasting period. 0 calories is your goal
- Always keep yourself hydrated with plenty of water (or tea/coffee/0-calorie drinks)
- Be aware if you take supplements, as some contain calories (especially those containing fats, i.e. omega 3, oils, etc.) so take them when you're not fasting
- Aim for 1 or 2 meals during your eating window
- Cut the snacks

As you can see, this IF plan is not difficult, in fact it's so simple even a caveman could (and did) do it – and you're smarter and more evolved than a caveman, right? #YabbaDabbaDoIt

The 50% Plan

Sometimes known as: Alternate Day
Brief summary: Eat "normally" for 1 day, eat 500-600 calories the next, alternate continuously.

The 50% Plan isn't what most people imagine when someone talks about fasting. Combining the principles of fasting with good, old-fashioned calorific restriction, this plan is very different to the Full-Timer Plan, and whilst it might not be the best solution for some, it will work brilliantly for others. This plan is especially good for those people who might struggle with extended periods of water-fasting (people who naturally suffer low energy, faintness, low blood-pressure and all that kinda stuff).

How to do the 50% Plan
So, again, before you begin using this plan, you need to know whether it's the right plan for you. Like I said before, one size does not fit all! If this plan seems to fit you better, have a go at it. Maybe you're not quite ready to jump straight into the Full-Timer Plan yet, if so, this is a great starting point to help you to make your mind up (hence the name).

Once you've thought about it extensively, weighed up all your options (perhaps gone back to the coffee-enema idea, briefly), and now you're 100% sure this is the right plan for you, you're going to need to think about how best to arrange the plan around your life, the universe and everything.

Obviously, being a one-day-on, one-day-off plan, it's tricky to keep your schedule exactly the same every week (seeing as there are only 7 days in a week, and we're working with an even-swap). Therefore, if you stick to the plan as it is set out, your weeks will alternate, looking something like this:

WEEK 1 STRUCTURE:

Mon	Fast
Tues	Eat Normally
Weds	Fast
Thurs	Eat Normally
Fri	Fast
Sat	Eat Normally
Sun	Fast

WEEK 2 STRUCTURE:

Mon	Eat Normally
Tues	Fast
Weds	Eat Normally
Thurs	Fast
Fri	Eat Normally
Sat	Fast
Sun	Eat Normally

If you would prefer your weeks to run in exactly the same way (you creature of habit you), then I recommend you structure your days thusly:

WEEK STRUCTURE:

Mon	Fast
Tues	Eat Normally
Weds	Fast
Thurs	Eat Normally
Fri	Fast
Sat	Fast
Sun	Eat Normally

Note: If you'd prefer to have your two consecutive fast days on different days, that's fine, this is just an example.

Obviously, with this structure you have two fast days in a row. It might happen that you end up with a distinct lack of energy on the second consecutive fast day. If this is the case, it may be worth either switching back to alternate days (suck it up), or you could add some extra calories for the second day, so instead of 600, ramp it up to 900 (this option is not ideal, however, as the 50% Plan relies on the fast days being around 20-25% of your normal daily calorific intake). Again, most people will be fine with the 2 consecutive fast days, but if it doesn't work for you, don't keep doing it (use your common sense).

"Can't I just have two Eat-Normally days instead?"
No. Do you want to lose weight or not?

OK, so what about the "fasting" part…
As mentioned, this plan doesn't use a true (water) fast, it is instead a modified calorific restriction fast. These fasts can take a little more getting used to than water-fasting, especially if you're going from having three "normal" meals a day (not to mention those filthy snacks you've been crammin' in yer mush), down to 600 calories per fast-day. 600 calories is not a large amount, especially if you try and split it into three meals.

Note: You probably noticed the "suggested calories" at the start of this chapter are 500-600. Remember, daily recommended calories for guys is around 2,500, and more like 2,000 for girls... So, following that logic, guys should have around 600 calories on their fast days, and 500 for girls. If you're a highly active female, then you may need that extra 100 calories, and if that's the case then OK, but only you can make that decision. Just don't lie to yourself. Going grocery shopping or vacuuming the cat doesn't count as "highly active". Also, the reverse is true; if you're a guy, and you're inactive, then you can probably do without the extra 100 calories. Don't lie to yourself.

For this plan, it's recommended that you use your calories in a maximum of two meals, the less "feeding times" the better (anything over three – including small meals/snacks – and your body can switch back to fat storing mode). Most people go for two, some will have just one meal, but you've got to remember that having just one meal can be a lot harder (psychologically), as it can feel a bit too "restrictive". It's also important to remember that you don't have to split your calories 50/50 over the two meals. So, one meal could be 500 calories, and the other could be 100, or 300/300, or however you'd prefer to balance the scales, so to speak. By eating two meals instead of one, you are also able to have more variety, and variety makes us happier than eating the same old thing over and over.

As with the Full-Timer Plan, you can have as much water, black tea/coffee or 0-calorie soft drinks as you like. Liquid is your friend, it will help you to feel full and will stave off any feelings of hunger that you might have. Hunger can initially be a bit of a bastard, but if you chug a glass of water, you'll generally find the hunger will disappear (or at least reduce) within a minute or so. Eventually it will barely even register at all.

Is meal timing important?
Unlike the Full-Timer Plan, it doesn't really matter when you eat your meals. If you'd like to experiment, you could work your fast days on the same principle as the Full-Timer Plan, and give yourself an 8-hour window to consume your 500-600 calories... Perhaps it would increase the benefits, but as with most things, if you don't try you'll never know. It's still worth noting that eating right before bed definitely isn't the smartest idea (it's generally best to leave at least an hour in between eating and going to bed), but otherwise, you have freedom to eat whenever you like. You can eat at the same time, or at different times every fast day if you want to. You could have breakfast and dinner one day, lunch and dinner the next, and just dinner and an early evening snack the day after, it's entirely up to you. The main take-home point is that you just have to ensure you keep below your 500/600 calorie target on fast days. It doesn't get much simpler than that!

Are there restrictions on what to eat?
The short answer is; no. This isn't a diet book, and
I'm not here to tell you what you should or shouldn't
eat, however there are certain tweaks you can make
on fast days to make this plan work better for you.
The best tip would be to aim for high-protein foods,
because protein is great at making us feel fuller
(...imagine trying to eat half a loaf of bread. That's
not *too much* of a challenge, I'm sure you'll agree.
Now imagine trying to eat the same sized half-loaf,
but this time it's made of thick, juicy beef steak... Not
gonna happen, because protein fills you up like a
boss!)

"What if I don't eat meat?"
If you're a vegetarian, firstly, wtf are you doing with
your life? (lol) Secondly, you are gonna have less
protein options, so you might want to stock up on
eggs, cheese, soy-products, nuts, beans, fish (if
you're a phoney-vegetarian who thinks fish aren't
animals), and some of that fake-meat stuff (that for
some reason is made to look as much like meat as
possible ...I never got the point of that). When it
comes down to it, whether you're a vegetarian,
pescatarian, omnivore or straight-up carnivore, you
can still use these fasting plans in the same way. It's
all good! #DefinitelyGoAndGetASteakThough #Nom

Moo-ving swiftly on...
Another great way to fill yourself up is to choose
high-fibre foods; whole-wheat bread and pasta,

brown rice, beans, nuts, pulses, dried fruit, bran, porridge, fruit and vegetables, etc. These foods are healthy *and* filling, and that's exactly what you want on fast days, because it'll make your life a helluva lot easier! Also, when you're taking in protein and fibre (mostly carbs), you're keeping the fat to a minimum.

Macros vs. calories
It's very useful to remember what each 'macronutrient' equates to in calorie terms:

Protein	=	4 calories per gram
Carbohydrates	=	4 calories per gram
Fat	=	9 calories per gram

Note: Alcohol = 7 calories per gram... just in case any of you drinkers were wondering.

Though fat is equally good at causing us to feel full, it's over double the number of calories per gram, which technically means you're able to eat over twice the amount of protein than fat, meaning you get more food for the same number of calories. You will appreciate this on your 600-calorie days! While we're on the subject of fat, obviously most "fast food" contains masses of the stuff, meaning super-high calories! As such, fast food is generally not the best choice to help you succeed with this plan. Here are a couple of examples of calorie content in fast foods vs. some relatively healthy foods, just to give you an idea of why eating a little healthier is probably a more sensible choice for your fasting days – keep in mind, you'll be aiming for 600 calories MAX on fast days:

Big Mac = 530 Calories
(Uh huh, and that's with no sides/drinks!)

Large French Fries = 510 Calories
(How do they get so many calories into a potato?!)

1 KFC Chicken Breast = 489 Calories
(Seriously, I'm not making this up!)

3 Slices Dominos Large Margarita Pizza = 580 Calories
(Holy frigging Jesus...that's with no toppings!)

VS.

200g Chicken Breast (roasted) = 180 Calories
(Less than half the KFC counterpart!)

60g Brown Rice = 220 Calories
(Super healthy, super filling!)

1 Cup Broccoli = 30 Calories
(30 calories? Give me 20 cups!)

Medium Egg = 60 Calories
(Clucking hell!)

1 Slice Brown/Whole-wheat Bread = 80 Calories
(A way better option than white bread!)

As you can see, you could eat 2 relatively healthy, filling meals; Egg on toast (no butter), and chicken, rice and broccoli, and consume less calories (570) than if you were to eat ¼ of a pizza (580) ...and honestly, can anyone really eat just 3 slices of a pizza??? I highly doubt it (...based on my extensive personal experience in this matter).

Now, if you had to eat the same small healthy meals *every single day* (like on many of the widely accepted diet options out there), perhaps you'd go crazy and give up within a week (I know I would). You'd probably also end up getting super run-down, due to not getting enough calories. With this plan, however, you get all the benefits of eating smaller, healthier meals, but without all the accompanying stress, deprivation (both physical and psychological) and associated negative emotions, because you don't have to do it *every day*, just every *other* day! Which makes this plan pretty awesome, right?

Note: It's advisable to have an idea (or a list) of possible low-calorie options that you can refer to when preparing your meals, because it's often really easy to over-shoot your calorie allowance by accident. If you want to learn more about foods/nutrition/meal-planning to go alongside any of these plans, then take a look at the "How to Eat Healthier" section towards the end of the book.

The "Fuck It" Moment
I went over this for the Full-Timer Plan, but I'm going to go over it again, and I'll go over it a third time for The Weekender Plan, because it's important. You are only human (unless there are any highly-trained service-dogs reading this, but for now, we'll assume you're human). As such, you are likely to have a slip up at some point. It's natural, it's normal, it's fine, just don't make a habit of it. If you want decent results then you have to keep at it, and I'm not saying it'll be super easy 100% of the time, but it sure as hell will be easier than most diets.

So, what if you accidentally eat 700 calories instead of 600 once a month? That's fine! But if you're having "fuck it" moments once, twice, three times a week, you're gonna get sloppy results. You'll soon get sick and tired of making hardly any progress, and you'll blame me and say that fasting doesn't work. Well it does work, unless *you* fuck it up...which I'm sure you won't, because I know just how much you want to ditch the fat, feel good and be generally an all-round awesome person! You have the abilities, you have the strength. Your focus determines your reality, so focus on your goals and let nothing stand in your way. #UseTheForce

"The 50% Plan" – Key Points:

- Alternate days, fasting and eating normally
- Eat 500-600 calories on fast days
- Aim for two meals max during your fast days
- Always keep yourself hydrated with plenty of water (or tea/coffee/0-calorie drinks)
- Cut the snacks

As you can see, this plan takes some conventional diet approaches, and makes them easier and more sustainable! #DisregardDiets #AcquireAesthetics

The Weekender Plan

Sometimes known as: 5:2
Brief summary: Eat "normally" for 5 days, eat 500-600 calories for 2 days, repeat.

The Weekender Plan is very similar to the 50% Plan, so this section is going to be way shorter as you basically already know this stuff...

This final plan is called The Weekender Plan because it's designed for people who can't handle the other two plans... wimps, as I like to call them (yeah, I said it, lol). All joking aside, this plan is great for all of you folks who have such drastically, mind-bendingly busy lives that your weekends (or whichever two consecutive days you're not working) are the only days that you are able to modify your hectic schedule. That said, I don't personally know very many people who are *truly* busy enough to warrant using this plan, because most people should be able to successfully incorporate the other two plans around almost any schedule. A lot of people are just too lazy or lacking in self-assurance to believe they can actually do the Full-Timer Plan or the 50% Plan, so they attempt to get by on the 'bare minimum' ...and the results are congruent with this.

Less investment = less return.

*Note: If it is literally impossible for you to undertake any other plan, or if the others are too 'intense' for you, then don't worry, it's better to do **something** than just doing nothing and remaining overweight and unhappy, right?!*

Right.

How to do The Weekender Plan

Once again, before you begin you need to make sure this is the right plan for you, yadda yadda yadda and all that jazz. This plan is super easy to fit around most lifestyles, because it's just two days a week, which is great for "ease of use", but not so brilliant for effectiveness. Now, I'm not saying this plan sucks, because it doesn't; if the only plan you are able to work into your life is this one, it's 100% better than doing no fasting plan at all, but your progress will probably be markedly slower than the progress of the folks using the other two plans, because they're able to commit loads more of their time to the goal of fasting, becoming leaner, and generally winning at life. #YOLO #WhoEvenSaysYOLOAnymore

With the Weekender Plan you are able to keep your weeks practically identical. You don't have to choose to fast at the weekend, if you'd prefer a Mon-Tues or Fri-Sat fast, or whatever, either way. As with most of this stuff, it's up to you to decide how best to work it around your life! Here's a rough weekly plan, if you

62

haven't managed to figure out what it looks like already:

WEEK STRUCTURE:

Mon	Eat Normally
Tues	Eat Normally
Weds	Eat Normally
Thurs	Eat Normally
Fri	Eat Normally
Sat	Fast
Sun	Fast

Again, with this plan you're gonna have two fast days in a row. So, if you end up with low energy on the second consecutive fast day, you're probably just gonna have to suck it up, because with this plan, the whole point is that you have the two days in a row to compensate for your five days of eating regular shit like a regular-shit-eater.

Note. As I continue to read what I write, I come ever closer to seriously considering a career in poetry. Dante Alighieri eat your heart out! lol

As with the 50% Plan, this plan relies on you eating just 500-600 calories on your fast days. The same principles also apply to meal timing, etc. and there's no point in me duplicating information and making you read the same things over and over again, now is there? So, if you need a refresher, head back to the 50% Plan to get the rub.

The "Fuck It" Moment

With this plan, it stands to reason that you should have a lot less "fuck it" moments, because this plan is a lot easier than the other plans and considering you're only gonna be spending two days a week fasting, you'll have a lot of time to blow off steam by eating "normally". I'd like to urge you to consider that your "fuck it" moments are more likely to come during the non-fasting periods whilst using this plan, because if you know you're supposed to be fasting on Saturday and Sunday, you could end up overcompensating, and making stupid choices on a Friday night...

Again, you get out what you put in. The odd pizza, though ill-advised, isn't gonna screw up your progress too much, but if you say "fuck it, I'm fasting at the weekend, so I'll have a pizza every night, and a burger for lunch every day, and hey, I'll have a double stack of pancakes with bacon and maple syrup for breakfast on Tuesdays and Thursdays too" ...well, at that point you're setting yourself up to screw yourself right in the fat ass that you *chose* to create! I know you don't want that, so just remember that you're 100% in charge of the plumpness of that ass of yours... It's entirely possible for you to get the sexy ass that you desire, but only if you remember not to "fuck it" too often!

#I'mNotActuallyTalkingAboutButtsexHere

"The Weekender Plan" – Key Points:

- Eat normally for five days, fast for two consecutive days
- Eat 500-600 calories on fast days
- Aim for two meals max during your fast days
- Always keep yourself hydrated with plenty of water (or tea/coffee/0-calorie drinks)
- Cut the snacks
- Aim to keep your non-fast-day diet a little healthier

To fast, or not to fast? That's not even the question. #JustPoetThings #RoryZShakespeare

Long Fasting – A Serious Warning

Although it might seem like a good idea to extend your period of fasting, you may actually do more damage than good. Some people like to do long/extended water fasts (where the only thing consumed over a period of 2-10+ days is water), but I would highly recommend that you do not attempt this. Although you would burn fat, the longer you fast, the more you would also begin to burn protein (muscle) too, and though that doesn't sound too bad on the face of it, you must remember that it's not just your abs, pecs and biceps that are made of muscle, your heart and organs are muscles too, and could also begin to deteriorate on a long-fast, resulting in the possibility of heart-failure (and you definitely *do not* want that).

Another risk of long-fasting is that of infectious disease. During a long water fast, your body will be starved of nutrients, meaning if you do get sick your body won't have the necessary energy to fight the infection, which can lead to dramatic complications. The ultimate (and obvious) risk that you face when undertaking a long-fast is death, and this has been known to happen in as little as a couple of weeks.

By undertaking a long-fast, the results could be dramatic but, at the same time, they can also be fleeting. Many people who try a long-fast will often go straight back to eating a load of crap (being "fed up" all day) after the fast, and consequently will regain all of the weight that they lost during the fast (and perhaps more besides). Fasting is best used as a long-term supplement to your lifestyle, because yo-yo dieting is not good for you, and long-fasting as a standalone method would fall under that category.

A useful thing to mention here is the principle of "Hormesis" which basically means you are given an ultra-small dose of something that in a larger dose would cause you stress/pain/death, this is done as a protective measure and is usually applied to diseases and viruses. This principle is used extensively in medicine and is known as: "vaccination". Yes, the basic principle of vaccination is very similar to those of intermittent fasting; a little "stress" on your system will actually give you a benefit, but if you have too high a "dosage" it may well screw you up.

Also, it has been known for people to become addicted to fasting, some due to the idea of "self-punishment" others due to the feeling that accompanies a long-fast (sometimes known as a "fasting high"), as with *anything*, fasting can be abused, over-used and taken to dangerous extremes.

Stick with the tried-and-tested plans, especially if you want to succeed in keeping the weight off, whilst staying healthy! If you're doing the Full-Timer Plan, cap your fast at 23 hours MAX! If you eventually decide that you want to have a go at a long fast (which again, I highly recommend against), then you should first seek advice from your doctor/physician and arrange for constant medical supervision during the fast itself – do not just "have a go" and attempt a long fast on your own, as it can be dangerous, and even deadly!

Extra Tips

So, we've gone through the plans, the science, the benefits, and by now you should (I hope) have some kind of idea about which plan suits you best, and when you're going to implement it (ASAP, right?). But the book's not finished yet...far from it, so grab yourself a 0-calorie beverage and get comfy!

This section contains a bunch of fasting hints and tips that will help you to more easily achieve your goal of losing excess body fat and becoming happier and healthier. Some of these tips are about useful things you can do, others contain advice about things that it'd probably be better if you didn't do, but all are designed to help make your life as simple as humanly possible during your fasting process!

Firstly, and most importantly we're going to talk about progress, because whichever plan you choose, it's going to be pretty important that you keep an eye on your progress. You're gonna want to check in with yourself frequently and evaluate how you're doing... So, how do we do that? Jump straight on the weighing scales? Actually, no!

Don't weigh yourself all the time!
Getting obsessed over the numbers on your weighing scales is stupid, boring and a complete waste of time and energy. If you weigh yourself and you find you've dropped a bit of weight, it's great, you feel amazing,

everything is good! That doesn't *always* happen though, and if you jump on the scales and you're the same weight as 2 days ago, or god-forbid, you *put on* half a pound ...OMG life is over! Screw this fasting lark, it can't be working! Give me a chocolate cake every hour, on the hour, and then I'll feel better!

...OK, so maybe it's not *that* extreme, but daily (and even weekly) weigh-ins are absolutely unnecessary for the vast majority of people. Unless you're entering yourself into a sporting event, and you need to weigh a certain amount to fit into your weight-class, ditch the scales. There are much better ways to check if you're making progress, such as; do your clothes still fit? If they're loose, you're making progress (and may need to buy new clothes soon).

Another great way to check your progress is to *look in a mirror*! Take off your clothes (all of them) and stand your butt-naked self in front of a full-length mirror. How are you looking? Generally, there will be 3 answers to this question:

1: "I'm still looking fat"
That's fine, because fat-loss (especially with large amounts of excess fat) will take time, so maybe don't expect a six pack within the first couple of weeks!

2: "I'm actually looking a bit leaner than before"
Awesome, then you need to keep going until you reach:

3: "I look fucking spectacular"
(I will also accept: "I have reached my goal", lol)
At this point, it's either time to re-evaluate your plan
for maintenance, or you can just carry on as you are.

Those are pretty much the 3 things you need to
"measure". You don't need to know if you lost a third
of a pound in one day, that information is
insignificant and it's totally boring! Have you ever
listened to someone whining about the miniscule
shifts in their body weight? It gets pretty old, pretty
fast, so don't be that guy… or girl… or transgender
person… or Helisexual (Google it, lol).

Also, by looking at yourself in the mirror, you are
giving yourself some amazing motivation right there!
I know so many fat, lazy people who choose to not
look in the mirror… Why? Because it makes them
feel bad when they have to look at their own fat,
naked bodies! No one wants to feel bad, let alone
about themselves. I've been fat too, and sure, when
you're fat, looking in the mirror sucks, but at the
same time, it's a great motivator …and I'll tell you
what sucks more than looking at your own fat ass in
the mirror; Being. Fucking. Fat! #TrueStoryBro

If you look at yourself in the mirror every day, front
view and side on, you'll get to learn what your body
looks like, and when you start making progress with
your chosen plan, you'll much more easily notice
how different you look with less fat.

Looking in the mirror at your excess fat gives you a physical enemy, your arch-nemesis personified. Whether it's the beer-gut, the muffin-top, the chubby cheeks, the chafed red thighs, the puffiness, the cellulite... your fat is your enemy, and seeing your enemy gradually disappear into nothing day-by-day is one of the best feelings there is. Becoming a parent? Nah, getting lean and sexy feels 100 times better (and is way cheaper, lol).

Note: Also, if you aren't a parent yet, getting in shape might help you towards that goal too! Because being overweight can screw up your procreating abilities, it can screw up your baby's health, it can screw up the conception itself, and it can definitely screw up your chances of getting laid in the first place... Hey, just sayin'!

So, look in the mirror every day, I don't care if you don't *want* to, make yourself do it anyway. I'm no Nike spokesperson, but seriously; just do it! Get to know your enemy, then destroy it like Spiderman throwing Voldemort off the Death Star into the fires of Mount Doom, or whatever... #PopCulturePro #DownWithTheKids #GetYourBirthdaySuitOn

Get some evidence!
Another great way to keep a check on your progress is to evidence the process, right from the start (and throughout). The very best way for you to do this is to take some photographs of your body. By taking

your progress photos, you'll be giving yourself the most accurate comparison possible, also you'll be giving yourself a truck-load of motivation, because comparing your progress photos to your start photo is VERY satisfying (trust me).

Another great reason to take progress photos is that you're always gonna have a picture of yourself from "back when you were fat", and it's probably gonna look pretty shitty, so in the future you can look back at that photo to remind yourself how far you've come. Now, if that's not motivation to keep yourself on track, then I don't know what is!

*Note: Obviously you might not want to do your photos butt-naked, just in case they fall into the wrong hands (and trust me, nobody wants to see your naked ass leaked onto the internet ...yet). So, I recommend that you strip down to underwear-only to take your photos. Also, if you keep the photos "safe for work" then once you've reached your goal weight, you can even send a before/after comparison in to me, so I can share it on **Hypno-Fasting.com** to show the world how amazing you are!*

There are certain considerations you need to remember when taking your photos. Location is important. You need to take your progress photos in exactly the same location every time. The location of where you stand and also the location of the camera need to be the same, so you can get an accurate comparison (because obviously, if you're closer to the camera, you'll look bigger, and vice versa).

The lighting needs to be the same. Don't use a flash on some pictures and not on others. Don't have the lights off, or the curtains closed on one, and not on another. Your aim is to keep these pictures exactly the same (or as close as you can get them), so that the only thing that will be changing is you! Always take your pictures at the same time of day, I suggest in the morning when you wake up, before you've eaten and after you've been to the bathroom (you'll learn to love how good your body looks after you've had a poop… weird but true). #JustTellingItHowItIs

There are 2 "poses" that you should do in these photos; straight on (facing your entire body directly at the camera) and side on (turning your entire body 90° so you're "side on" to the camera). Now, it should go without saying, but *don't* "suck it in", because if you breathe in to make your stomach look smaller, the only person you're cheating is yourself. Let it all hang out! Yeah it might not be pretty at first, but the worse it is, the better your motivation (and the more awesome your comparison pictures are going to be later on).

Taking your photo(s) once every two weeks or once a month (if you can wait) is generally about as often as you'll need to do it. Any more frequently, and you won't be seeing *as much* progress and you may "de-motivate" yourself, so there's no point!

Do you measure up?

Get yourself a tape measure (preferably a sewing tape measure, which you can pick up almost anywhere for next to nothing). Use this tape measure to wrap around various parts of your body to check your measurements. You *could* measure your waist (where your belt goes), but I find measuring around the stomach (over the belly button) a much more effective motivator and indicator of progress. You can also measure other parts of your body, your upper arms, your thighs, your ass, etc. (as we don't tend to store all of our excess fat in just one place, and each of us stores fat differently).

I don't know if I need to say it, but I'm going to anyway; when you measure, don't pull the tape measure tighter to make the number smaller, it doesn't work like that! It needs to be an honest measurement, not pulled tight, and make sure that you measure around the widest area. If your tape measure isn't big enough, buy another one and tape 'em together, then try again.

It can be a good idea to take your measurements at the same time as you're taking your progress photos. Once you've written down your measurements with the date, you can take a photo of that too, then you've got the photos, the measurement and the date all in one neat, handy pile. I know, I know… you can thank me later.

Dear Diary…
Some people like to write a diary to document their process. The two main things that you might want to cover in the diary, would be your thoughts about the fasting process/the progress you're making, and food information. Writing down *everything* you eat in a diary is a great way to keep yourself accountable, and to check and see if you've been lying to yourself and overeating. Also, I've said it already, but you've got to remember; drinks often contain calories too!

If you think you might use a progress diary, you can also use it as a place to write down your body-measurements, and you can even stick your progress photos in there too, if you can be bothered to download them and print them out (because I over-confidently assume you won't be using a Polaroid camera).

Anyway, these are 4 of the most effective ways to keep tabs on your progress, and if you only do one of them (looking in the mirror is mandatory, so that doesn't count), then make it the progress-photos, because they are a seriously useful tool for measuring progress and boosting motivation. So, now we've covered how to track your progress, let's take a look at some other stuff…

Give it time to get used to the plan

As with most change, it may take you a little while to get used to fasting. That's perfectly normal, so chill Winston. Remember back near the start of the book I mentioned how little time it can take for a new habit to be formed? Well that's good news, right? In a matter of weeks your new eating habit will become something that you just do. It'll become something that you barely even need to think about, because habits are pretty easy to create, so long as you stick with it. We all make mistakes, have slip-ups and "fuck it" moments, but if you are as consistent as you can possibly be, the habit-building process will be a lot quicker and a lot easier.

Don't punish yourself if you have a "fuck it" moment

We've covered the "fuck it" moments with each plan, and as I've said; we all do it! If you don't have "fuck it" moments then you might be a robot, so I'm gonna hide my clothes... my boots... and my motorcycle (#ArnieWouldBeProud). So, if you say "fuck it" once in a while, don't beat yourself up. If, however, you say "fuck it" more often than not, then you might want to re-evaluate which eating plan is best for you...or be a little stricter with yourself. You've gotta commit to succeed!

Don't pig out straight after a fast (save it for later)

Though it might be tempting to "make up for lost time" by eating more than you normally would, straight after your fast (or on a non-fast day), don't. Just don't. Start off with a regular meal (or perhaps even a small one) and enjoy having a little restraint.

Note: If you're 330lbs or something, and your "regular meal" is an entire family bucket of fried chicken, 4 servings of fries and a bottle of Pepsi, then you might want to change your idea of what a regular-human-sized portion is. Eating enough food to feed a family of 4 in one fell swoop is not a regular meal. You cannot fast away that kind of excess and gluttony. #SozAgain

Binge eating is unnecessary and unhealthy for humans. You don't need to eat thousands and thousands of calories in one hit, you're not a Reticulated Python! Eating too much food in one go will stretch out your stomach, therefore giving you the ability to eat more and feel less full – this will definitely not help you in any way whatsoever.

What will happen if you go "Yeah, I had an awesome 16-hour fast and I feel leaner already. NOW GIVE ME THAT WHOLE FAMILY SIZED PIZZA! OF COURSE I WANT FRIES TOO! NOM NOM NOM!"?

...well, you'll feel fat, bloated and crap! Bingeing may make you *think* you "feel good" temporarily, but in the long-term it's gonna make you feel a whole lot worse, both physically and emotionally.

Stick to "normal" portion sizes when possible. What's a normal portion size? Ball your hand up into a fist... Your clenched fist is (generally) about the same size as your stomach, so if the mass of food on your plate is much greater than the mass of your clenched fist, then you're probably overeating. As with all of this, you don't have to take my advice, it's not mandatory, but if you want to lose some fat, and want to make decent progress, then it may be worth taking some of these points into consideration...

Choose what you want to eat
Obviously on the Full-Timer Plan you can choose to eat whatever you want, but also, if you've chosen to use one of the calorie restriction plans (50% Plan/Weekender Plan) then you *still* get to be creative with what you eat. You can choose exactly what foods will make up your daily calories, there are absolutely no restrictions on what you're allowed to eat (in fact, restrictions would be a terrible idea), so you can enjoy choosing what you're going to eat on your fast days, but just remember, a small amount of "unhealthy food" is generally going to contain a lot more calories than the same amount of "healthy food". Hence, if you want to feel fuller for less calories, the healthy option is often the smarter option. For instance: 1 "large" serving of french fries from a fast food restaurant contains about the same number of calories as 11 large whole cucumbers. Do you think you could eat 11 whole cucumbers in one sitting? If so, that's impressive, but I doubt it.

So, you can eat more of the healthier stuff, or you can eat less of the unhealthy crap... it's entirely up to you! Quite frankly, after a couple of days of eating just 1 portion of french fries for a whole day, I'd be quickly re-evaluating my meal choices to get the most out of them! Just a thought...

"Is this plan a long-term, sustainable solution?"
Hell yes! You can continue to easily and successfully use any of these fasting plans long-term. You can safely use them *forever* if you want to. If you keep to the plan for a long time, you will eventually reach your natural limit, where your body will be lean, your blood-sugar control will be awesome, you'll be the master of your hunger, and cravings will be a distant memory. Once you get to this stage, you'll be able to easily maintain your bodyweight, and because your body will be great at using fuel efficiently, you'll be able to eat a bit more and fast a bit less.

Some people (those who've reached their natural limit with fasting) continue to get all the benefits of fasting whilst only actually having to fast for one or two days a week. So, unlike other diets, the longer you do this, the easier it gets! Ain't that just the icing on the cake!

Always respect/pay attention to your body
Throughout this entire fasting process (and preferably during the rest of your life), you should be listening to what your body is telling you, because

your body often knows what's best. If there's something wrong with your body, then generally something needs to change. As I've already said, if you're under lots of stress already (too much exercise, not enough sleep, too much alcohol, drugs and all that kind of stuff), then starting a fasting plan might not be the most sensible idea, and you might end up stressing your body out even further! Don't do that, it's not worth the risk.

You must respect your body, because you only get the one (well, until they start growing replacement limbs and organs ...which will probably happen sooner than we expect), but for now, if you don't respect your body, you pay the price. We've all had a friend or relative who we've loaned our precious belongings to, only to get them back all scraped, smashed and fucked up. Now, would you loan your *body* to that person? Probably not. So why would you mistreat it yourself? Bottom line is: pay attention, and if your body is trying to tell you something is wrong, take immediate action to figure out what it is and change what isn't working for you.

Feeling Hungry?
Talking of paying attention to your body, let's talk about hunger. Just because you *think* you're hungry doesn't always mean you actually are. There is a huge difference between psychological hunger ("head hunger") and physical hunger ("true hunger"). Head hunger is frequently the result of boredom,

habit, stress or chemical cravings. Perhaps you might recognise yourself in one of the following situations...

Picture the scene:

You got home from work, had your evening meal and sat down to watch a little TV. The food you ate 20 minutes ago has barely begun to digest but, damn it, this TV show just isn't the same without the sound of yourself chomping on a pack of Doritos or a tub of Ben & Jerry's. Oh, and then there's the subsequent thirst, which of course you must cure with a tasty alcoholic beverage (or five) because that'll also help you to "unwind" after a stressful day at work...

or

You get in your car and set off on a 2-hour round-trip to pick up a second-hand exercise bike (to help you get in shape), that you found after trawling through pages and pages of inappropriate sexual posts on Craigslist. But, yeesh, you forgot how boring this whole driving thing could be, and to top it off, your radio is broken too. So, what could possibly help make this arduous, dismal challenge of an expedition into something a little more bearable? Hmmm... a drive-thru snack of course! Fuck it, you're in the car already, right? Might as well occupy your mind by filling your face-hole (...good job you don't think the same way about your other holes, you dirty food slut)!

or

You go to the movies with a friend, you buy a huge box of popcorn and your friend buys a big family-sized bag of chocolate treats. They then decide they don't want it and donate it to you... You know you don't *need* them, as you already finished the popcorn before the movie even started, but once you've eaten one piece you find that you just can't stop (that'd be the serotonin release, which is a chemical that induces a temporary state of happiness). "Yay, nom, nom, nom, nom, oh wait I'm starting to feel sick, let's ignore it, nom, nom, nom, nom, urghhhhh I ate too much again..."

If you could see yourself doing any of those things (or maybe something similar, but perhaps a little less extreme) then well done, you're human. As a human, many of us have learned to think that "head hunger" means that we're hungry. Luckily for us, as humans, we are able to re-program the way that we respond to such things.

Fasting is a great way to re-calibrate our hunger-sensors. By sticking consistently to your fasting plan, you will naturally overcome the old bad habit of listening to your head hunger. By doing this, you will naturally learn what your true sense of hunger feels like, and that can only be a good thing for your appetite, your weight, and your overall health and wellbeing.

That said, even if it *does* turn out that you are in a state of "true hunger" it doesn't mean you *must* eat immediately. Hunger is not the master of the faster! As you find your fasts becoming easier (and they do), the easier you will find it to notice your hunger, acknowledge it, and then put it out of your mind because you want to fast for another hour or two.

Hunger is nothing to be afraid of, in fact it is something to be embraced. Hunger makes us feel alive, alert and energetic (as mentioned previously; when our bodies are hungry, our minds go into "hunter mode" and give us more energy and brainpower). So, embrace the hunger! You might even learn to love it! #NoPromisesThough

Give yourself time to overcome cravings
Cravings come and go, and they usually don't last for very long at all. Whenever you're fasting and you find yourself thinking about eating something, have a drink of water and busy yourself with something else (anything else) instead. Drinking a large glass of water helps by making you feel less "empty" and will cause the feelings of hunger to diminish. After having a drink of water, you will usually notice that the thing you were craving doesn't actually seem as important, and you can then continue being absolutely freaking awesome, and you'll more easily finish your fast.

Even without the water trick, if you are "craving" something, anything, don't immediately give in to your impulses. Make yourself wait for 20-30 minutes. Anyone can wait for 20 minutes, and by simply doing that, you'll usually knock that internal feeling on the head ...and that's all it is, a feeling, it's not an addiction-craving, you are not *addicted* to cakes, ice cream, biscuits or chips, so "reframe" the way you refer to these *feelings*. Your mind is a powerful thing and can be used to help make fasting much easier!

Idle hands do the Devil's work ...and the Devil is probably a fat guy

It's a great idea to keep yourself occupied during your fast. If you're sitting about doing sweet FA, then you'll have plenty of time to think of all the things that you *could be doing* to easily alleviate your boredom, such as; seeing how many Snickers Bars you could fit in your mouth... making an XXXL pizza with 50 different toppings... eating a deep-fried stick of butter with a knife and fork... This is not the type of stuff that you want to be thinking about. Thinking food-related thoughts will not help you to achieve your fasting goals, and more to the point, it will make you feel like shit too! So, what can we do about it?

If you're fasting on a "work day" then you shouldn't really have too much free time anyway (unless you're the obligatory lazy person in your own work place). Work should be keeping you too occupied to think about eating, and if it doesn't, you might need to start working harder! Also, by doing more work to keep your mind occupied, you might get yourself a promotion, earn more money, etc. (a win-win situation, I think you'll agree).

What about the days that you're not working? Well, the simple answer is; go and do something! Here's a list of things that you can do, instead of sitting on your ass thinking about food:

- Visit your family/friends (they might appreciate it!)
- Watch a movie (...and remember that you don't need snacks in order to do this!)
- Read a book (Never read one? Well the dictionary is a good starting point)
- Write a book (Well, if I can do it, anyone can!)
- Talk to children (preferably your own!)
- Pre-prepare a load of healthy meals to freeze and store (more on that later...)
- Masturbate (hey, we all do it ...right? lol)
- Fuck your partner (it's the one type of cardio that anyone can enjoy!)
- Fuck someone else's partner (running away = extra cardio)
- Clean your car
- Play a computer game
- Go for a walk/bike ride and look at some nature-stuff
- Write a to-do list/bucket list (and then go and do the things that you wrote!)
- Take up a new hobby (swimming, fishing, stamp collecting, art, anything)

- Clean your house
- Start an argument with a street-preacher (it's not hard, trust me)
- Become one with the universe
- Jump to conclusions
- Go for a walk, and pretend you lost your dog/child/senile grandparent
- Search for buried treasure
- Pretend you're a tree for an hour (see if you can communicate with other trees)
- Do something interesting/odd, record it, stick it on YouTube and become an overnight internet sensation

Disclaimer: I am not responsible for anything that happens if you do any of the weird examples I just suggested.

The opportunities to fill your time productively(?) are endless – remember, we only have one chance here on this big spinning ball of earth and water hurtling through the universe at 67,000mph, so you might as well do some of the things that you want to do, and have some fun whilst you're here (and if you can lose weight at the same time, then that's a bonus)!

Modern life never stops
Some people have the opposite problem where there is always too much to do, and not enough time to do it in. Just because you're busy, it isn't an excuse to eat crap and snack all day long. You'll probably

find that by fasting you free up a little more time to get stuff done, which might in turn provide you with a little "free time" every day where you can just chill out, even if it's just taking a few minutes to yourself, sitting down, closing your eyes and relaxing.

Note: Taking just 5 minutes out of your day to relax can make your entire day better, so if you're always busy, stick a note in your diary to give yourself a break! The less stressed you can become, the more likely you are to succeed with your fat-loss goals!

Fasting doesn't make you die
This point is kind of unrelated to everything else, so I just decided to stick it in here... lol

I have had people ask/state: "If I don't eat for a day, surely I'll die?!" – This (supposedly serious) question is often asked by people with no fasting experience (and nay-sayers). Sure, if you miss *all of your meals* and eat absolutely nothing for days and weeks on end, then yeah, you'll probably die, but you're not gonna die if you miss a meal each day! If you use these fasting plans every day for the rest of your life, you'll probably actually live *longer*. Like I said before, fasting is good for you.

Focus on the quality of the process, it's sometimes more important than the outcome
Fasting is a great way to lose fat, but there are a couple more awesome benefits that you can

experience when using a fasting plan:

- You learn to respect eating
- You learn how to exercise self-control
- You can learn more about how your own body works
- You learn from experiencing true hunger, and how it represents itself to you
- You can enjoy taking a break from preparing so much food
- You can enjoy taking a break from feeling obliged to eat
- You can enjoy using your time more productively
- You can enjoy knowing you're privileged enough to choose not to eat
- You can enjoy pushing yourself (safely) past your pre-conceived limits
- ...and obviously, you can lose some fat too!

So, by using **Hypno-Fasting** you're effectively learning more about how to work alongside your body, thoughts and feelings. You're developing self-control, you're freeing up more time to use for whatever you like, you're coming to terms with the idea that you do lead a positive, privileged life, you're learning that you can surpass your own limitations... Holy shit, that's a lot of added benefits! They should teach fasting in schools (...I definitely shouldn't be the teacher though). #A-IsForApple #B-IsForBoobs #YouAllKnowWhat-C-IsFor

Get support
No, I don't mean buy a bra (...unless you have moobs, then it might save you from some awkward chafing). Having support, for *some* people, can be the difference between success and failure or happiness and feeling like a big steaming pile of poop. Here's a little exercise for you, and all I'd like you to do is use your imagination... I'd like you to imagine for a moment, that you're the type of person who needs/prefers to have support... and also imagine that you are a closet homosexual. Imagine that you really want to tell your friends and family that you're gay, but you don't think they will support you in your decision, so you decide to keep your sexuality "in the closet". Imagine how that would feel... Pretty damn bad, right? (p.s. if that's *actually* the case, maybe get new friends who aren't douchebags).

Now, I'd like you to imagine the same scenario, except this time Imagine that you *do* have the support of all your friends and your family... With that powerful feeling of support behind you, imagine how much easier it would be to "come out". You could pounce out of the closet like a sparkling, fabulous unicorn escaping from Narnia, and you'd be happy with your life-decision, because the people that matter to you are on your side!

Yes, sometimes support makes things a lot easier, and it's true that some people feel the need for additional support, whilst others don't. Some of you will *naturally* be like those brave, fabulous unicorns throughout every aspect of your lives, without even trying, without ever seeking approval, or needing other people to tell you that "you can do it" or "you're strong enough" or "you're doing the right thing, by making yourself happy". Other people, however, might need encouragement, enforcement, accountability and support... and that's fine too!

If you don't have people around you in "the real world" who can give you support, go out and find other people who are in the same boat as you. Well, I say "go out" but in the age of smart phones and internets and moveable print, who needs to go out any more? Go online and search for other people who are just starting out with fasting, write a blog, post your progress on forums, use social media, etc. On Facebook alone, there are thousands and thousands of special interest groups and forums, you can even join the **Hypno-Fasting** Facebook group:

Facebook.com/groups/hypnofasting

...feel free to post there and tell your story, support each other, share before & after progress photos and all that kind of fun internetty stuff!

Anyway, what I'm saying is, even if support is not "readily available" (i.e. family and friends), there are still going to be support-channels available to you, if you're willing to put in a little leg-work and find them. One thing I will say is, just make sure the people giving you support are actually committed to helping you become happier, healthier and a better person, because people can be weird...

Some people may appear supportive, when in fact they're actually trying to sabotage your progress. Yes, there are many douchebags out there, and yes, sometimes the douchebags might be closer to you than you can imagine, so be careful, because a lot of people suck (and I don't mean in a sparkly, emo vampire kinda way)!

If I want your opinion, I'll ask for it! But I won't. Following on neatly from that last point, let's talk about people who will do exactly the opposite of support you. Now, hopefully you won't have to deal with too much of that, but if you do, best to be forewarned and forearmed, right? You may hear all sorts of negative (or "concerned") comments, like:

> "You're doing what? Why the
> hell would you do that?"

> "That sounds dangerous...
> You might get sick!"

> "You've gotta have breakfast, it's the
> most important meal of the day!"

"You're upsetting me by doing this."

"WTF that's stupid bro, drink your protein shake, think about the GAINZ!"

"That's a fad diet, you're stupid."

"Derp de derp 3 meals a day de derp…"

People can be very negative, sometimes excessively so. They can distrust, discourage and fundamentally disagree with anything they don't perceive as being normal or accepted. They can do this without even knowing what they're talking about. They can do it without knowing your motivations. Hell, sometimes they can just do it for fun, or to piss you off. You need to train yourself to not care what these negative douchenozzles think, because caring about what they think won't help you in any way whatsoever.

As you saw a moment ago in the list of things people might say to you, some of these things won't be out-and-out negative. Sometimes people are very sneaky about delivering their negativity/disapproval in a way that creeps under the radar, by making it appear "compassionate" or "concerned". Sure, you can be worried about someone's health, but as the person who's fasting, you're in control of your fasting-related-health, and if anything negative were to come of fasting, you'd be the first one to hold your hands up and say "OK, that's not working for me, I'll stop". What you don't need is someone wrongly assuming that fasting is unhealthy when it isn't, and trying to convince you to stop it, right?

Whether negative, disapproving or even faux-compassionate, you can approach these types of question/statement with logical responses, and hopefully the person in question will accept that you're old enough to make your own decisions and life choices. Hopefully they will listen, and perhaps, just perhaps, they will realise that you are actively improving yourself, and they may even champion you for it and give you encouragement... Sometimes, however, they won't. Sometimes, just the simple fact that you are trying to make yourself better will piss them off immensely. This may be because they don't have the guts or the willpower to do the same kind of thing for themselves, or maybe they're just inherently a douchebag on a cellular level. Who knows? Either way, if you encounter a person like this who won't be reasoned with, you're probably not going to convert them with words. Change the subject, and next time they ask, just tell them that you're eating normally again (if you must). When, weeks or months down the line, they notice your progress and they see that you're a lean, mean fat-burning machine, they may be amazed... They may even want to "know your secret" ...and that's the perfect time to rub it in their whiny douchebag faces and tell them to go violate themselves with a cactus (or, you know, have a normal polite conversation with them… your choice). #CactusForTheWin

You obviously don't want to upset your family or friends, so you must play it by ear. So, don't upset them, but also don't let them stop you from doing what you need to do. Find a way to work around their questions. Find a way to work your eating plan so they have less cause to ask about it. Always eat with your family at night? Well make that your main mealtime. Always visit your grandmother on a Saturday? Well make that one of the days where you can eat "normally" (because as we all know, refusing food from a grandmother is definitely not advisable – you don't wanna screw with granny)!

Eventually, as I said, people are going to see your results, and the nay-sayers may even ask you for advice on how they can "shed a couple of pounds". Actions (and results) speak louder than words, but you must always stay true to what *you* want to do, regardless of what other people think. Just make sure you don't make life unnecessarily hard for yourself while you're doing it.

What if I want to give up?
If you get to a certain point where you are feeling the "fuck it" vibe more and more often, and constantly thinking "man, I want to give up" then I highly recommend that you just give up. Don't keep ploughing away at something that isn't working for

you! I bet you weren't expecting me to say that, were you?

Note: Wanting to give up in the first couple of days/ weeks doesn't count. Sack up and stick to the plan!

Honestly though, if you eventually find that you've lost your motivation to stick to the plan, or to actually achieve your goal, then don't force yourself. Quit (or take a break), find out why you've lost your motivation, re-think things, and then, when you're ready, you can start again. Sometimes things only need a little adjustment to make them work better, so perhaps make a couple of little changes before you jack the whole thing in completely.

Before you give up, ask yourself why you are giving up. Don't just quit for some BS reason, like: "hmmm, I miss breakfast cereal" ...that's ridiculous (and is probably your sneaky mind trying to trick you to regain "normality", like I mentioned before).

I frequently come across people who say they want to quit because they're "not losing any weight", but in most cases, when questioned, it turns out they've been eating like 500-1000+ calories more than their fast day allowance, or their daily 8 hour eating window had become more like 12-14 hours. If that's the case then you might as well quit, because it ain't gonna work if you're not gonna put in the effort and follow the plan.

So, if you need a break, or need to make some changes to make it work better for you, then by all means do it. We're all different, and obviously it's a good idea to make things work for you, rather than forcing yourself to work around something that doesn't.

The plans in this book are pretty universal, and *most* people will be able to fit them into their schedules, somehow, or at some point (if you've got too much stuff going on in your life, then come back to it when you can fully commit).

Commit when you're ready to commit and ready to change, but make sure that when you do, you commit fully and completely! Don't half-ass it, because if you half-ass it, you're gonna see poor results, make limited progress, feel like crap, and give up anyway. So, give yourself the best chance to do well. Be like a parrot and suck-seed. #Succeed #DadJoke #YourJokesAreBadAndYouShouldFeelBad

Programming Your Mind for Success

This section is all about helping you to become better at fasting and sticking to your chosen plan until you reach your goal. I've split it up into 3 key areas. Firstly, we're going to look at some common, unhelpful thoughts and beliefs relating to food and eating. After that, we'll come onto a whole bunch of information about how we (humans) work psychologically and how aspects of our psychology can be used in order to make the fasting process easier (as well as some cool "mind tricks" relating to eating). The final section is all about motivation and includes some great tips on how you can keep your motivation levels high, how to ensure you're able to fully commit to your fasting plan, how to set your weight loss goals effectively, and how to stop yourself from getting in your own way (which we're all guilty of, in one area of our lives or another).

Note: Many of the key points in this section are covered (in one way or another) within the hypnosis MP3 download that's included with this book. I'll talk about that at the end of the chapter, because it's important that you read this section before you listen to the MP3, so that you can fully understand and engage with the MP3 for your best success.

Thoughts and beliefs

We each have many different beliefs about food and eating, some healthy, some less so. Some of our beliefs are, in reality, downright ridiculous, but they're *our beliefs*, which means no matter how ridiculous or technically inaccurate they are, *we* still *believe* them to be true! That's what a belief is. So, if you have any beliefs about food/eating that you think could be holding you back, it's a good idea to "challenge" said beliefs. We'll go into that in more detail in a little while, after we have covered some of the most common beliefs that limit (in some way) the success of people who're trying to lose weight (no matter what the diet/plan).

Free food

Who can resist free food? Free food is all over the place, you can get free samples at the supermarket, people you work with may bring food in for everyone to share (whether on a daily basis, or for staff birthdays and special occasions), hell, sometimes people walk down the street with free samples of food. It can be anywhere, at any time, and hey, might as well, right?

...*no*, and I'll tell you why...

Free food, unfortunately, doesn't tend to "register" in our minds as being "food" or counting to our daily calorific intake. This is similar to snacking, the logic behind snacking being "it's not a meal, so it doesn't count", but it *does count*, calorie-wise. When people snack on free food, they don't modify the rest of their daily intake to factor in what they've already eaten for free, which means the calories begin to add up and up. So, just because you *could* eat as much free food as you like (and not suffer financially for it), doesn't mean you necessarily should. To draw an analogy, imagine having a serious romantic partner, a girlfriend/boyfriend/husband/wife (or think about your actual one). Now, in this example, your partner is your "daily meals". So, imagine going into a shop, and having someone offer you "no strings attached sex for five minutes" would that count as another "meal"? Or because it's only very brief (and free), does that mean it doesn't count at all? Would it be worth that tiny amount of (potential) enjoyment, for the sake of the long-term repercussions? I say "potential" enjoyment, because you never know what that free food (or sex) is going to be like... It could be entirely mediocre and pointless... It could be absolutely gross... It *could even* make you sick (yes, all of these examples could apply to either food or sex, lol) ...but because it's free, fuck it! Might as well have a go, because it's there for the taking. Can you see how this might be an unhealthy, unmindful way of getting through your day/life?

Challenge the belief: Whenever you are presented with an opportunity for free food, why not take a brief moment to ask yourself one very simple question: "If this thing wasn't free, would I actually, actively want it/pay for it/get it myself right now?" if the answer is no, then you know what you need to do. Don't cheat on your meals, they have feelings too you know!

Cheap food, deals and buying in bulk
So, you've gone shopping. You've bought lots of nice, healthy foods …but then you notice one of your old staple "treat foods" is on sale, 3 for the price of 1! You had no intention of buying this item, but it's 3 for the price of 1, goddamn it! So, you ended up buying three of the things you didn't even want to buy one of in the first place. But why? Marketing is why! You got sold to. Large companies who sell food don't tend to care about whether you're trying to cut down your calories, because they are more interested in you buying their products. #OhTheHumanity #OrMaybeNot

If you have more food readily available to you, you'll generally tend to eat more on a daily basis. If you have multipacks and family bags and 50% extra's, you're likely to continue eating (or drinking) those things beyond the time you would've if there was a smaller amount available to you.

Challenge the belief: Yes, buying in bulk technically makes things cheaper in the long run, but it's unlikely that your purchases will be *used* in "the long run", so in fact you're paying more *and* using more. If it's an offer on something that you had already *planned* to buy, and it's "buy one and get the second half price", you're only saving 25% off each thing, *but* you're still spending an extra 50% more than you would have if you'd not been a victim of marketing (or if you'd not been greedy), and if you had just gotten the one. When you find a deal, ask yourself honestly whether you actually *need* more than you'd initially intended to buy, so that you can make the right decision.

As well as special offers and deals, sometimes the people who serve you/take your order will try to "up-sell" and "on-sell" to you, this is their job. They are another group of people who really aren't bothered by your calorie intake, but only the takings of their business. So, they *want* you to "go large" or "supersize it" and have an XL coke instead of a medium. If you were going to order a medium then order a fucking medium. Are you that suggestible that you'll buy *anything* just because you'd already chosen to buy *something*? (If so, I offer private 1-on-1 **Hypno-Fasting** mentoring for just $5,000 per hour, it's literally a steal, contact me for details, lol). The same goes for "on-selling", just because you bought a cup of coffee, doesn't mean that you can't resist when the girl at the checkout says "oh, would you like a pastry with that coffee?" – *learn to say no*. People that can't say no to anything are often not healthy, not happy and not in control of their lives. Is that you? Start now, by saying: No! Hell, even say no to my request that you start saying no, it's a start! lol

Wasting food

"There are kids starving in Africa, clean your plate" we were told as children. Don't leave food on your plate, you're lucky enough to have all the food you could eat, so eat all of the food that we give you. A nice way to ensure your child gets enough fuel and nutrition, but also a great way of installing a sense of guilt, an over-eating habit and an unhealthy belief that we *must* clean our plates, even if we're full and there's still food left. It's not just *our own plates* either; for those of you who are parents of children who *don't* heed the "children in Africa advice", there are even more plates that need to be cleared! ...and it's much better for that cold, half-eaten, drool-covered child's food to go into an already-full parent than into the trash, right?! ...guess what...

WRONG! Lol

Challenge the belief: No matter whether you choose to put the excess food into your stomach or throw it in the bin, either option means you will not be helping any poor, starving African children in any way whatsoever. Yes, you may feel "less guilty" by not wasting food, but how guilty will you then feel (when you evaluate what you just did), and you realise that you bought and ate way more food than you actually needed? That you may have even eaten so much that you made yourself feel sick, when you could have comfortably eaten perhaps 25% less? Will you then feel guilty knowing that you could have taken that 25% of your food bill and donated it to savethechildren.org or unicef.org and *actually helped some starving children*? Or will the guilt come when you realise that obviously you're bothered by starving children (enough to cause yourself to be physically and emotionally uncomfortable at mealtimes), yet instead of help them, you still choose to stuff yourself full of food excessively until you feel like shit?

And breathe... no one said challenging long-held, unhealthy, unhelpful beliefs would be easy or fun. I'm just making a point here, that sometimes our beliefs are skewed or faulty. What *we* eat doesn't directly correlate to starving children. Wasting food doesn't have to be about starving children at all. Sometimes it's just that we just don't want to "throw money away". If something's going out of date tomorrow, let it, and ditch it, because it's better to bin the food rather than eating it (on top of your normal meals) just because it's going out of date. Other times, we'll buy something new to try, find out we don't like it, but then force ourselves to eat it anyway because we paid for it. That's about as smart as buying some underwear, finding out later that it is 5 sizes too small (and uncomfortable in naughty areas), but going ahead and wearing it anyway because you've paid for it. A pretty stupid idea, right? So, have a go at throwing stuff away that you don't want or need, it can be quite liberating. Also, work on changing your shopping list, recipes and portion sizes so that this issue doesn't come about in the first place. If you're a parent, and your kid doesn't often finish his/her meals, give them a smaller portion, and if they're still hungry after, give them dessert or a snack, it's a win-win for all involved.

Have you forgiven me for the African children yet? :-)

Politeness (a distinctly British problem)
We, as decent folks, have a tendency for politeness. Some of us are *way too polite* for our own goods, actually putting the emotions and feelings of others above our own physical health and emotional wellbeing. Making ourselves feel crap, all in the name of politeness, or not wanting to hurt people's feelings. Let's say your lovely old grandma baked a bunch of cupcakes for you and your family, and she slaved in the kitchen with her bad back and gammy leg for hours to make these lovely treats for you all. If you were to refuse it, that would make you a terrible person... right?

Not quite...

Challenge the belief: Food does not equal love. Giving food *can* be a token of affection, sure, but refusing it does not mean you hate, loathe and despise the giver. If your alcoholic uncle (who you love dearly, and worry for his health) asked you to sit with him and drink a bottle of whisky each, would you decline? ...I assume yes, but what's the difference? He could be upset that you're refusing his "kind gesture", and you might actually like the whisky equally as much (or as little) as your gran's cupcakes (they both contain lots of calories). But wait, let me get this straight, you love your uncle, and want him to stop drinking *for his health*, but you also love granny, and want to eat her baked goods *regardless of your own health*... Something doesn't quite add up here, does it?

I know it sounds trite and cliched, but in these situations, you need to remember to love yourself (not literally, lol). No, you need to think of yourself as one of your loved ones. Would you force granny to eat some unhealthy food you made, if you knew she was trying to lose weight and improve herself? No... that would be a dick move. Maybe granny knows you're trying to lose weight and would like to help, but she just can't get past the whole "granny must feed everyone" factor, or perhaps she thinks she knows best ...but she isn't you. *You* know what's best for you, and you know that the best way forwards in this kind of situation is to acknowledge your desire to please the people you love, but to favour your desire to do what's right for you. Care for yourself as much as you care about the feelings of your family, friends and colleagues. Put yourself first once in a while.

So, you pretty much have 2 ways around the "eating out of politeness" dilemma. Option 1 is to be direct, explain to granny that as much as you'd love one (and really appreciate that she made them, and they look great, etc.), you're currently working on improving yourself and doing something to make you happier and healthier, and that you hope she can respect that and help you. It can also be worth mentioning that it won't be a permanent thing, so you *will* be able to eat her foodie-gifts again in the future, once you've met your goal. Do this respectfully, and most people will accept and allow it (yes, even granny). Option 2 is to thank granny, and tell her you're too full right now, or that you have a bit of a stomach ache, but you'll take a serving and eat it later (and then, when you leave, throw it away, or put it in the dog, or a friend, or something else). It may seem "mean", but with option 2 everyone is happy ...even the dog. #BeMeanGetLean

I deserve to treat myself
We often have busy lives, and some of our lives are harder than others. Not everyone has the best support structures or the healthiest reward-strategies, but commonly with people who are overweight, food can be thought of as a reward, a coping strategy, or quite simply, just a way to make ourselves feel better. Food is easy to get, plentiful, and does "the job" fast. The problem is, when you are emotionally motivated towards eating (i.e. for a reward/support), the food choices you're likely to make won't tend to be very healthy. Often this can come down to speed and ease of use. It's super quick

to just open a bag of something fatty and calorific to reward your own "successes", or to microwave something ready-made in a futile attempt to dampen your heightened emotions. Speed of creation, however, is not often a key factor in the creation of truly delicious foods, so are you *really* treating yourself to something amazing, or are you just shoving something easy and mediocre down your throat?

Challenge the belief: Food is nice, I'm not going to disagree, but there's a big difference between choosing to eat something because you want to and eating due to a compulsion. You may have decided to believe that, because you parked your car 3 spaces further away from the supermarket entrance, that you deserve a whole chocolate gateau as a reward for "upping your exercise". You may have gotten into a pattern of stuffing down your negative emotions using chocolate biscuits, using whole packs at a time to cram that emotion back down into the pit of your stomach... However, when you think about it logically, would *you* be as forgiving to someone who did the same thing, squashing their emotions down, but instead of food, they used excessive amounts of alcohol, or maybe even drugs? Because that's what you're doing when you're emotionally eating, you're abusing substances in an unhealthy way to mask your emotions. Perhaps a great reward for hitting your target at work would be to go and treat yourself to an evening with a hooker (it doesn't matter that you have a partner at home, because this is just a "special reward" because you "deserve it"). See what I'm getting at?

Sure, you have needs. You have the need to feel good emotionally, but you also have more needs, needs that are less related to your instant emotional gratification (or emotional suppression). You can reward yourself in other, less damaging ways. What makes you happy outside of food? What is a treat or a pleasure to do? Perhaps you enjoy reading, so make it your treat to spend that money that you may have spent on a pizza, on a new book to enjoy, or a movie, or go out and do something fun, hang out with someone you like. Food is just food, it's not a trophy, and it's also not a therapist. If you're having trouble with unhelpful emotions, negative and unwanted feelings, then perhaps you owe it to yourself to do something about it... Talk to a trusted friend or colleague, go to your doctor/GP and ask them for help, or seek out counsel from a third-party professional. Eating won't make hurt go away, in fact it can make it worse, as well as causing various other problems along the way.

Life is boring without food (and drink)
Going to the cinema ...gotta have popcorn and sweet things! Going for a coffee ...gotta have a cake with it, or my coffee will just be too dull! Having a cup of tea with the family ...must have some biscuits for dunking (may just be a British thing, lol). Meeting

with friends for a catch-up …alcohol and snacks are a given. Drinking wine …can't have wine without cheese and crackers. Drinking beer …pizza or kebabs are mandatory. Road trip …can't drive more than a few miles without having my driving-nibbles to keep me occupied… yadda, yadda, yadda.

Challenge the belief: Most of the time, the things that we're doing *are* entertaining enough to keep us occupied without needing to add food or drink (or alcohol) into the equation. Going to see a movie is a form of entertainment in and of itself, mindless eating does not increase the entertainment value of the movie experience, because, for the most part, you're just shovelling food into your face and not paying attention to what it tastes like anyway. The "food = entertainment" idea basically boils down to a form of psychological conditioning. A "conditioned response" is something that can happen when we combine some activity with eating. So, say we do something a few times in the same way (such as, buying popcorn each time we went to the movies), and we also manage to attach a positive association to the link (such as by telling ourselves "this is fun" each time), then, with repetition, this new way of doing things becomes a habitual, unconscious process. So, once the conditioned response is in place, we go to the movies and we're on autopilot when we say; "a ticket to Ghostbusters and a large popcorn please" (the original Ghostbusters, not the remake, obviously). Our mind loves shortcuts, and it loves them so much that it can convince us that our *learned* way of doing things is the *only* way of doing things – anything else is "just not fun".

If the things that we do aren't fun, it's highly likely that we wouldn't want to do them in the first place. If you didn't want to hang out with your friends, go to see a movie, read a book, socialise with your family, go to a coffee shop, etc. then you'd probably choose not to do those things. So, it's time to re-acquaint yourself with the things you do and why you do them, *without* the associated conditioned-food-responses. Change your routine. Do your stuff and enjoy doing it for the right reasons. Engage with the movie fully, take some water in with you in case you're thirsty, eat before you go so you don't get hungry, because if you're not hungry, you don't eat. Enjoy and savour the things that you enjoy, without needing to "on-sell" yourself to having extra things to stop yourself from "being bored". Do something different or active with your friends and family, go shopping, go for a walk, go to the beach... You're in that situation *for* entertainment, so pay attention to the situation and enjoy the entertainment value.

If you still think the food/drink is making the situation more entertaining, do this simple test: take the same food/drink (same type and same amount) that you'd have in that situation, take it home, sit at a table in a room all by yourself, doing nothing else, no TV, no music, no people, no other distractions, and eat/drink the whole lot in one sitting. Once you're done, rate the entire experience on a scale of 1-10 for "entertainment value". It's very likely that this thing you're doing "for entertainment" isn't actually that engaging or entertaining at all. In fact, it's probably pretty boring by itself.

So now we've covered things that are fundamentally entertaining, what about the stuff that isn't? Sometimes we *have to* do things, things that we may not want to do, so it's important to remember something that, in this day-and-age of technology and instant gratification, we may have forgotten; not everything is *supposed* to be interesting or entertaining. Some things you just have to do... Suck it up! So, you're bored? Oh no... Just because wittle baby is a teensy-weensy bit bored, doesn't mean you need to cram shit in your face-hole, does it? If you can't hang out with your friends without binge eating crap or drinking booze, maybe you need to re-evaluate why you hang out with these friends... are they friends, or are they an excuse for you to go off the rails and not feel bad about it?

Boring things are boring – eating won't help.

Entertaining things are entertaining – eating won't change that.

Be mindful of why you're doing what you're doing, and if you think you might be doing something for the wrong reasons, or because you've conditioned yourself into an unhealthy habit, then have a word with yourself and challenge your own reasons and beliefs for *why* you're doing those things.

How to challenge unhealthy beliefs
So, we've briefly covered some of the common unhealthy/unhelpful beliefs around eating, however you may have *different* beliefs (or different versions of some of the previous examples), so it's important for you to learn that you can challenge your beliefs, and to know that just because something has been a belief of yours for a long time (or even for as long as you can remember), that doesn't mean you don't have the ability to change your beliefs, because we all have the ability to change our beliefs when we need to ...if we want to.

Imagine you were taught to play poker by a friend (who didn't quite know all of the rules). Sure, you got on OK in games at home with your friends, but when you decided to take a trip to the casino for a "real game", you came to realise that your beliefs about how to play poker weren't actually as true or effective as they could have been, and maybe you got confused... maybe you got some strange looks from the other players... maybe you even lost some money... But, do you then quit poker *altogether*, just because of these old beliefs? No, of course not, because you enjoy poker. So, instead, you decide to read a book and look online to learn *a better way* to play the game. You have come to realise that the way you've been doing things for years (based on your initial experience and continued reinforcement) was not helpful in the long run, even if it did help you initially play poker with your friends. So, you have chosen to change your beliefs, by challenging them against facts, and by looking at the situation objectively, rather than assuming that the old way is the right way, without having any *real evidence* to back up that old set of beliefs. You know that just because "that's the way it's always been" doesn't necessarily mean that's the way it *should* always be, and yes, it may be tricky at first, adapting to these new beliefs (the old way *was* so familiar to you, and therefore easier), but by persisting you'll gradually learn how to play poker properly, and you'll come to realise just how much more effective you can be, simply by challenging that old belief, and accepting that change.

So, before we go over some ways that you can do this, first we have to get to the bottom of the belief itself. What is an unhealthy/unhelpful belief that you have? Ask yourself (and answer honestly) about the *belief* behind your behaviour, such as:

If you're emotional eating, why?

If you're eating for a reward, why?

If you're eating for another reason, why?

If you're eating for no reason, why?

If you're eating more than you know you need, why?

If you're worried about wasting food, why?

If life is boring without food, why?

Whatever your belief is, you'll need to question it, and once you've answered, then you may need to get to the bottom of *that* answer. So, you may need to question your answer(s) too. As an example:

You think life is boring without food, why?
"Life is boring without food, because I don't have anyone to hang out with"

...why?
"um, because I'm not confident enough to go out and socialise"

...why?
"I guess because I had a bad breakup, and I never got over it"

...that's just a potential example (and could go on even longer, or in any direction), but it's worth knowing that the beliefs behind your behaviours can sometimes be complex and linked to other things, and yet, at other times they may be ridiculously straight forward.

Once you have your belief(s) written down (I've provided a box below for you to write them down as you question and challenge them), then it'll be time to move forward in the belief-challenging process:

What's your belief? Question it.
What's your answer? Question it (and repeat if needed).

So, from that exercise, you should get your core belief, or, "the main thought" that this whole thing boils down to. Getting to that core belief can *sometimes* be tricky, and it might take a couple of attempts, it might take a bit of deep thought and a hefty dash of honesty, but if you give it your best shot you'll get there, because *you know you* better than anyone else does.

Once you have whittled your beliefs down to that one "main thought", it's highly likely that it will be some kind of belief about yourself, such as:

"I'm... X"

"I can't... X"

"I should be able to... X"

So now it's time to challenge the belief. You're going to have to do the work, because just reading these next couple of paragraphs isn't going to do it for you. Once you understand the process, *do the process*! The easiest way to challenge a belief is to question it. Put your belief on trial and see how it holds up. Where is the evidence that proves it is true? Is it logical, if so how? How would it help you if you were to continue believing this? What are the benefits of keeping this belief vs. the costs? Ask all of those questions, challenge every aspect of the belief, and accept that, sometimes, your answers may surprise you. When this happens, take a moment to really think about what that answer means. Engage fully with any answers that come up, and connect to what that means for you *now,* and how changing that belief could then positively impact your life

If you struggle with those direct challenging questions, then it can be helpful to change your perspective in order to continue, and there are a couple of ways to do this. Imagine you found out that a friend of yours had your belief, your exact belief/situation, and they were saying something similar to themselves, what would you say to them? Another way to shift your perspective is to imagine explaining your situation (and your beliefs) to 100 random people, what would they think about it? Would they think your rationale was correct or faulty? What kinds of things would 100 random, unbiased people say about your belief? Sometimes, we need to get out of our own way in order to accept new (challenging) information, and a third-party perspective (or a hundred third-party perspectives) can be very useful.

A final way to help you get out of your own way, is to imagine that your belief (and the corresponding behaviour) is like a dream. When you're asleep, your dreams become your complete and total reality, you *believe* everything that's happening is true... is fact... simply because you're experiencing it. *This* dream *seems* completely real, but when you awaken from this dream, it begins to fade, and you realise that you can see it from a different perspective now. A few moments ago, it felt so real, so all-encompassing, so true... Yet now, you're awake. You still remember what it was like to have been inside that belief, inside that dream, yet you understand that all it was, was a collection of thoughts and ideas. This knowledge can allow you to let go of any fear that you may have had before, when you were asleep, when you were dreaming, because you know that now you're awake, things have changed.

Do this: Take a deep breath in now, and hold it... Then when you're ready, exhale and relax...

So, you've challenged your belief (and if you haven't, feel free to do it now, and come back to this point when you're done). Now, if you could replace your old belief with another healthier, more helpful belief or thought, what would you prefer it to be? Maybe you can find a healthier "preference"... So, if your belief is; "I must have a bar of chocolate after a hard day at work to relax" perhaps instead it could be; "I'd prefer to have some chocolate after a hard day at work, but I know there are many other ways to relax too". Changing your belief from a demand (must) to a preference gives you an option, it gives you flexibility and choices. You deserve to have flexibility, happiness, healthiness and control over your own behaviours. The old unhealthy, unhelpful belief was rigid and immovable, *making* you do things that you didn't really want or need to do. It's nice to have some "wiggle room", and to be able to exercise your freedom of choice. Accept now, that though part of you might feel like it "must carry on as you always have", that there's a new part of you that would *prefer* to move onwards in a slightly different direction...that would prefer to make choices rather than always doing the same thing over and over like a broken record. It's time to change the record.

Note: For those of you who are young, "records" are what people listened to music on before tapes, CDs, MP3 Downloads, YouTube and Spotify. #RetroAsFuck #TheMoreYouKnow

Psychological eating tactics

There are many, many psychological tweaks we can make to "trick ourselves" into doing things, especially when it comes to food and eating. They're not all as simple as getting a child to eat with; "here comes the airplane!" ...but some of them aren't far off (and sometimes the easy solutions are the best)!

Actively question your eating process

Let's say you fancied a sweet snack, so you grabbed a bag of sweets or chocolates out of the kitchen and proceeded to eat the whole lot over a period of ten minutes. It's likely that you thoroughly enjoyed the first couple that you ate, but it's also likely that your enjoyment begun to taper off with each successive one that you ate, until you ended up just eating for the sake of eating, or eating mindlessly. I cover this particular topic again in the "How to Eat Healthier" section, but with a slightly different focus.

Fundamentally, you need to ask yourself why you're eating, or why you're continuing to eat. If you fancy a sweet snack, you must remember at the outset that a snack is not a meal, so the key thing you're eating for in this case is pleasure, not quantity or nutrition. If you're snacking, stop yourself a few mouthfuls in and ask yourself honestly; "do I need any more of this right now? Am I enjoying it as much now? Have I got what I wanted already?" ...you probably got what you wanted after a few mouthfuls. Sometimes less is more.

Imagine you get to eat a delicious, gourmet meal. Then imagine that you have to eat the same gourmet meal every day, for every meal. Initially it would be amazing and a real delicious treat, but after a few days, *because* you'd been eating it constantly, you'd be bored of it. It would still be the same delicious treat food, but it would have lost most of its "treat appeal". It'd become more of a mindless habit, or something that you have to just "get through" until it's gone. So, make sure your treats remain treats, enjoy them, savour them, be mindful of eating them and totally connect to the experience of eating them. Stop eating them once you feel that you've enjoyed enough to class it as a treat ...maybe not just 1 square of chocolate from the bar, but perhaps not all 20 of them! You shouldn't be eating treats in order to "feel full". If feeling full *is* what you want, then there are healthier, less-calorific food choices that will help you to do this... but if you don't ask yourself the question initially, then you'll never know why you're eating

Whenever you're just about to grab something to snack on, or something to drink, imagine that you've got a remote control with one button on it, the PAUSE button. So, when you're reaching for something to put in your mouth, hit PAUSE, and take a moment to think and question your process. Imagine doing it now, going to the kitchen and grabbing your favourite dessert/snack... hit PAUSE. Question your eating process. Imagine doing this for a moment for your main, go-to snack foods. Run through the process in your head, over and over, but each time, imagine hitting that PAUSE button to give yourself the opportunity to evaluate what you're doing, before you choose whether or not to go ahead. When asked to make a big decision, people often "need time to think about it", but this principle can apply to smaller decisions too. Perhaps you could even hit PAUSE and go and do something else, then come back to your decision 10 minutes later... you may find you've changed your mind completely.

At some point, you might find yourself standing in the kitchen, and you can't decide what you want, or even if you actually want to eat anything at all. Maybe you're just bored, or craving "something". If this happens, all you need to do is ask yourself one simple question; "would I eat an apple right now?" ...if the answer is yes, then you're probably actually hungry, so feel free to eat something (it doesn't have to be an apple, but if you can't decide what to eat, PAUSE and come back to it). If the answer is no, you wouldn't eat an apple, then you're not hungry, so have a drink of water and go and do something else.

Note: If you don't eat apples, replace "apple" with a fruit or vegetable that you do like.

Emotional eating
Whilst questioning your eating process, you may find
that you're eating because you're feeling emotional.
You may be feeling down, and so choosing to eat to
get the *brief* release of positive chemicals
(dopamine) that unhealthy foods give you. But those
feelings don't last, and they will never deal with the
emotion itself – junk food is not the edible
equivalent of a therapy session, sorry. If you realise
that you're an emotional eater, firstly you might like
to go back to the beliefs section and go through that
process with your emotional eating related beliefs.
Secondly, you might want to think of other ways to
healthily subdue said unhelpful emotions. If you
want a quick release of natural, feel-good chemicals,
exercising is a much better choice (and creates a
longer lasting release of endorphins). Other things
such as, engaging with hobbies, reading books,
watching TV shows or movies, meditation, etc. can
also help to replace eating as an emotional coping
strategy. Often, however, the most effective course
of action is when you can commit to dealing with the
emotions themselves. Now, sometimes this will
mean seeking outside help, and whether that's going
to see a doctor, therapist or counsellor, or perhaps
confiding in a friend and asking for help, whatever is
easiest for *you* to accomplish is the best first step.
Sometimes you might need to take more than one
step, and that's fine too, because so long as you can
find a way to help yourself to become healthier, then
the "label" of how you get help is less important. Put

yourself and your health first, and remember, health doesn't just mean fitness, your mental and emotional health is equally important.

Distracted vs. mindful eating

So, you've realised you may be eating too much, and know that you need to question your eating process… but what if you're distracted? "Binge eating" (eating without thinking, in large amounts) happens most frequently due to distractions. So, this one's simple to fix, all you need to do is follow this one instruction; *only eat in designated eating areas*. If you eat whilst watching TV, stop it. Only eat in the kitchen/dining room. If you take a pack of Maltesers into the bath with you, stop it. Only eat in the kitchen/dining room. If you eat whilst reading a book… well, you get the idea. Be present whilst eating, and you'll easily stop any mindless, distracted binge eating. Remember, we don't need food to make things fun!

Mindfulness simply means "being in the moment", so to eat mindfully all you need to do is focus on what you're doing. Focus on your eating process. Focus on how your food looks, smells and tastes. Focus on the texture of the food in your mouth, the feeling as you chew, the feeling as you swallow and how it feels as it travels through your body. Each time you take a bite of food, count the number of times you chew (it should be around 15+ per mouthful). If you notice you are having other

thoughts whilst eating, acknowledge that you're having other thoughts, and then go back to paying attention to what and how you're eating. When you do this, you will find that your food tastes better, you will also find that you feel fuller sooner, and that you can actually notice when you are full and stop eating …even if there's food left on the plate.
#RememberTheAfricanChildren

Have a plan
It's said that "if you fail to plan, you plan to fail", and this can be a useful thing to keep in mind. Having a meal-plan can help you to avoid making rash decisions about what to eat. Another aspect of an effective meal-planning process is the shopping part, i.e. the part where you gather the ingredients that your meal-plan consists of. Shop around your meal-plan, and only buy the things that you actually need to make those meals. If you have low self-control (or are easily sold to), maybe switch to online shopping/ grocery deliveries, so that you are not confronted with special offer signs, enticing smells, salesmen and free samples… Also, go shopping after you've had a main meal (yes, even if you're shopping online), so that you're not making food purchases on an empty stomach, because if you do, you *will* buy more crap that you don't need. That's a fact.

Planning doesn't just apply to meals either, you can also plan your snacks and treats. Perhaps you have a "craving" for something… a useful way to put these cravings out of your mind is to let yourself know that you *will* be allowed to have the thing that you're craving, but you just have to wait until your allotted time. So rather than grazing on crap all day, you'll know that after your evening meal you can have your cake and eat it too (in moderation, remember). This helps to free up your mind for the rest of the day from thinking about things that you want to eat, because you know you'll get to eat what you want later on. Remember, treats are called treats for a reason. You can always have more another night, your favourite treat is not going to cease to exist overnight, so chillax!

Eating with your eyes

Your eyes can play a big part in your fasting success. It may sound strange, but a big part of feeling satisfied when eating is the visual aspect. A full plate of food is a piece of information that we see, and interpret to mean "oh good, we will be full soon". A great way to trick the eyes/mind into the same response, but to save some calories, is to simply use a smaller plate. It's still a *full* plate, it's just a different size – and size doesn't matter (in this instance, lol). So, if you use big plates and bowls at home, go and invest in some smaller ones. Also, if you eat food "on the go" and use containers or Tupperware, then clear/see-through containers work best, this is because you can actually see how much food you've got, and therefore you'll tend to eat less. The same goes for bags and packets of food, if you usually eat crisps/chips (out of a family-sized bag for instance), transfer some into a bowl. If you eat biscuits/cookies out of the pack, stick one or two on a plate, rather than taking the whole pack away with you. By "portioning" snacks out, you're still getting your snack, and when you finish your "portion", you'll probably feel just as satisfied as if you'd sat and eaten the whole lot.

Another thing relating to sight that can be applied to fasting for more success is the old adage of "out of sight, out of mind". If you don't have snacks and food out on the counter, or somewhere that's within your visual field, you're less likely to be reminded of food unnecessarily when you're going about your daily routines. We tend to arrange our lives (mostly) so that we need to think as little as possible about what we have to do, as such, we are generally able to create the conditions to make our lives easier. Make your life easier by taking food out of your vision, as much as possible.

Eating with your mind
Did you ever see the research about how "thinking about exercising" can produce real, tangible benefits? A group of people who sat and imagined themselves exercising had a notable increase in strength/muscle in comparison to the control group. That was the actual result of a research study, and yes, the same principle can be applied to eating. Though it might sound strange, if you're feeling

hungry, imagining eating food can actually reduce your hunger and cravings. Now, when I say imagining, I don't mean just thinking about taking a bite of a food, you have to fully imagine eating, in as much detail as you can and in "real-time". Give yourself a couple of minutes, get comfy, close your eyes, and run through the entire process of getting/eating your chosen food. Imagine every aspect of it; going to the kitchen, choosing it, opening/preparing it, holding it in your hand (or on a fork), the smell, the taste, the feeling and textures as you eat, the act of swallowing, etc. By taking your time over this imagination-process and going through it in real-time, it will make it much more effective. You'll be sending signals to your brain that you're eating, and the brain will often respond to it almost as if you really were eating (just like with the exercise study). Give it a go the next time you want to extend your fast for a little while longer, you may be surprised at how well it can work.

Punctuate your eating session
If you finish reading a story, you know it's the end because it either says "The End", or the next page is blank. When you finish a TV show, you know it's done because the credits roll and the adverts come on. We like things to have a definitive ending, a "closing point", something that shows us that this thing we're doing has now finished. So, how do you know when you've finished eating? What's stopping you from continuing your eating session beyond this

meal, or beyond dessert, munching away into the night? A great way to end your day's eating is by brushing your teeth just after your evening meal. This is your "The End", it's your final exclamation mark at the end of the chapter. Once you've brushed your teeth, you have closed your "eating loop" for the day. You start by brushing your teeth, you eat throughout the day and end by brushing your teeth. We, as humans, love it when "loops" close, and if that closure doesn't happen, we get

...agitated. (I wasn't going to finish that sentence, to prove my point, but I figured I'd get emails telling me I'd made a typo, lol)

Eating with others
Another thing to keep in mind that can drastically alter the amount of food we eat is whether we are eating by ourselves or with others. It's said that if you eat with someone else, you're likely to eat between 30-50% more food than you'd have eaten if you were eating alone. This percentage can change depending both on the number of people in your eating group, the people themselves, and the occasion. If it's a larger group (let's say 8), and it's a special occasion, it's likely that you could even end up eating up to 95% more than you ordinarily would! So, though there's only 8 of you, the bill may read more like a table of 16! This relates neatly in with two of the previous sections that we've covered; eating whilst distracted, and "politeness" (read:

social compliance). So, if you're eating with friends or family, just remember that you don't *have to* have a 3-course meal if you'd prefer just a main course (even if everyone else is having all 3), and also, just because you may be the first one to stop eating (when you're full), doesn't mean you *need* to keep eating until everyone else is done. If anyone questions it, feel free to tell them all about the African children… it always makes for a lively dinner conversation. #ConversationalistExtraordinaire

Remove your "trigger foods"

Warning: If you're squeamish, you'll hate this section (but it'll work even better).

If you have a type of food that you'd really like to stop eating, but you can't manage to do it by sheer willpower alone, then you can use a psychological technique known as aversion therapy. This basically consists of attaching a negative response to something that you want to stop having/doing. So, let's say you want to quit having crisps/chips… Think about some food/drink/substance that absolutely disgusts you, something you would really hate the taste of. For some people it's sprouts, for others it's Marmite, maybe even seafood… Whatever food you absolutely detest the smell/taste of. If you don't particularly have one, then think about something horrendous that you'd never want to put in your mouth (like runny, sloppy dog shit… or old man phlegm… or a 2-week-old used-tampon…) did that do the trick? (I did give you the warning at the start, lol). So, imagine the grossest thing you can… you can even combine a few, and imagine them in a bucket. Once you have the "aversive substance", I want you to then imagine taking the chips (or whatever you want to stop eating), and covering them in the gross substance… imagine that horrible bucket of gross, rancid crap, steaming and putrid… Imagine dipping a chip in it, swirling it around, so it's totally covered, and then imagine bringing that chip up to your mouth… smelling the stench of it… feeling the smell already clinging to the back of your nose and throat… then imagine putting it in your mouth, sitting it on your tongue, squelching and seeping as you chew it… trying not to vomit… the taste a thousand times worse than the horrendous smell…

Now stop. Clear your mind and take a deep refreshing breath of clean air… Shake it off, lol. Pretty gross right? Well, if you repeat this process in your imagination a number of times, and connect to it as vividly and completely as you possibly can, the more you do it, the more those chips will become associated with that horrible substance, and you'll begin to automatically react to the chips in a negative way, in the same way as if someone physically put that bucket in front of your face. This whole thing works on the premise of creating a "conditioned response" (Google "Pavlov's Dog" for more info on how this works psychologically). This is a tried-and-tested therapy technique, and one that hypnotherapists use frequently in their sessions (in fact, this technique alone helped me to quit my decade-long habit of nail-biting, in one session... so, it definitely works, and you can totally do it yourself, outside of hypnosis). You can do this either in your imagination, or you could even do it in real life, with the actual foods themselves. Obviously, only do this in real life if the gross substance is edible, non-toxic and you're not allergic to it, don't do it with spit and poop and sperm and puke and any of those things, that would be a bit silly and you'd probably get dysentery or something. Feel free, however, to dip your chosen food in other foods that you hate, and actually eat them, whilst telling yourself how gross and horrible the experience is. Maybe have a bucket ready just in case... and maybe don't do this technique if you have emetophobia (fear of vomiting), lol.

Sleep!
Though not an "eating tactic" per se, the fact is, if you're not sleeping well, your weight loss progress is going to stall or stop entirely. You need to sleep in order to lose weight effectively, and with a huge percentage of adults fitting into the "sleep deprived" category (something like over 30% of people), is it any wonder that people are struggling to lose weight and obesity is on the rise?

If you're getting less than 7 hours sleep per night, then it may be a good idea to work on sleeping better to support your fasting progress (also, added bonus; more time sleeping = less time fasting). It's generally recommended that between 7 and 9 hours is the optimal amount (varies slightly for each of us). Not getting enough sleep has (at least) 6 negative effects on weight loss:

- Increases your brain's need for food
- Increases Ghrelin production (which means we burn less calories/feel hungrier)
- Produces less Leptin (which makes our stomach feel empty)
- Makes us choose bigger portion sizes
- Makes sugary, high-fat foods seem more attractive
- Makes us too tired to exercise as effectively

So, as you can see, getting good sleep is a high priority for those who're looking to lose weight. Obviously, this book isn't about sleeping better, but there are some simple things you can do in order to get some good shut-eye:

- Turn off lights – darken your bedroom
- Turn off devices – blue light screens affect melatonin levels (sleep hormone)
- Put your alarm clock/phone out of sight/reach

- Ensure your mattress is less than 10 years old (or replace it)
- Anti-allergy bedding/reduce allergenics in bedroom
- Keep the bedroom for sleep and sex only
- Get into a bedtime routine (sets your body clock)
- Ditch the naps (save sleep for bedtime)
- Cut the caffeine (stimulant)
- Cut the nicotine (stimulant)
- Don't exercise too near bedtime (finish 3 hours before ideally)
- Don't eat too near bedtime (finish 2 hours before ideally)
- Cut the alcohol (it's bad for sleep quality, even though it may initially help you *get* to sleep easier)
- Don't drink too much water before bed (so you don't need to get up to pee)
- Know that sleeping tablets aren't a healthy, long-term option

If you've gone through this checklist and are still having issues with sleeping, it could be worth consulting your GP/doctor. I also have a free "hypnotherapy for insomnia" MP3 available, just search "Rory Z Insomnia" on YouTube to listen to that. #SweetDreams

Motivation, resource-building and other tips

So, we've looked into thoughts and beliefs, as well as some psychological eating tactics that can help you succeed, but what about if you want to improve your motivation to succeed in general? Perhaps you'd like more willpower, or internal resources... Well, there are a whole bunch of ways to both connect (or re-connect) to why you started fasting, and to help you keep engaged in order to reach your goals...

Goal Setting

If you really want to lose a certain amount of weight, however big or small the amount might be, then how about setting yourself some actual, tangible goals? Goal setting is a really useful tool to ensure that you stay motivated and continue to move in the right direction.

Now, when I say goals, I'm not talking about a broad goal such as; "I want to lose weight" because even though the end result that you're after is (sort of) there, it's not a well-thought-out goal. If your goal *was* "I want to lose weight", then you could lose just 1lb in 1 year, and that would mean you'd successfully achieved your goal, wouldn't it? Well, of course it wouldn't... 1lb in 1 year is terrible! ...but according to your initial goal, that would class as a success. See what I'm saying? With goals, you need to be specific, and to do that you can incorporate a couple of really useful goal-setting concepts, the first being; SMART goals.

SMART Goals are:
Specific
Measurable
Achievable
Realistic
Time-focused

You need to make your goal **specific**, so instead of "I'm going to lose weight" your goal could be "I'm going to lose 200lbs" (yeesh). OK, so you're going to lose 200lbs, but how will you know when you've done it? You need to be able to **measure** your success. So, take your weight at the very start of the process, on or before your first day of fasting (right now's fine, if you want to take a moment and get it done… I can wait). Then, once you start fasting, you need to continue to take measurements periodically (every couple of weeks/month) throughout the process until you reach your goal. Simple.

This goal that you're setting also needs to be **achievable**, which simply comes down to whether it is physically possible for you to actually achieve it. If you weigh 200lbs and your goal is to lose 160lbs, that is an unachievable goal, because if you somehow managed to get down to just 40lbs, you'd be pretty dead (maybe even very dead). So, your goal must actually be possible. If you have no idea what your end "goal weight" should be, Google; "how much should I weigh?" to get a rough idea.

OK, it's specific, measurable and achievable ...but is it a **realistic** goal? If your goal is unrealistic, the fact that you'll struggle to reach it will piss you off immeasurably, so make it something that you believe you'll actually be able to achieve in the time-frame that you're aiming for... So, following on from that point, your goal also needs to be **time-focused**. As mentioned, this *also* needs to be realistic, because if your goal is to lose 200lbs and you intend to do that in just 6 weeks, odds are fairly high that you're not going to achieve that goal, because in such a short time-frame it becomes highly un-realistic (or, in this 200lb example, *impossible*... even if you ate no food for 6 weeks, which you shouldn't, wouldn't, and couldn't, lol).

So, here's an example of a SMART goal using the 200lb example: "Today I am 380lbs. 2 years from today, I will be 200lbs lighter. I will know I have reached my goal because I will then weigh 180lbs."

Obviously, that's an extreme example (as 380lbs = 172KG = 27.1 stone), but it's probably not as extreme as you'd think, and is becoming ever more common, especially living in the western world). So, perhaps it might be better if the big end goal was broken down into smaller, more easily achievable chunks...

Chunking is basically taking your big goal/end result and turning it into a bunch of smaller goals that have shorter time-scales and are easier to achieve. This is a great way to keep your motivation up and makes your goal seem a lot more manageable. So, from the SMART goal mentioned before (200lbs), you could then chunk that down to a monthly level (using a calculator and some mathematical-wizardry) and your new shorter-term-goal would be: "I will lose 8lbs a month, every month for the next two years." By doing that, you then have a goal that is measurable every month, and if you went off track and only lost 6lbs in one month instead of 8lbs, you'd know that you would have to change something to meet your goal for the next month. You could chunk down even further to a weekly level (2lbs) if you wanted to.

Resisting change
It's important as well, when setting your goal, that you can actually "connect" with it, that you actually want it. It's also worth knowing whether any part of you *doesn't* want you to reach your goal (and this can sometimes happen without us even realising it). It's true that sometimes we do things that aren't healthy or helpful to us, because they serve a *different* purpose that *does* help us in some way. This is known as a "secondary gain". Here are a couple of examples that illustrate how some unhelpful/ unhealthy (bad) things, can actually serve a secondary helpful/useful (good) purpose:

A teenager smoking (=bad)
...in order to fit in with his friends (=good)

A woman overeating and gaining weight (=bad)
...in order to repel unwanted sexual advances from men (=good)

Someone having stress-related pain (=bad)
...that stops them having to lift a finger at work (=good)

Obviously, these "good" results are subjective (meaning they are specific to each person), and different people have different motivations for doing things. It's important to get an idea whether you have any "secondary gains" at the goal-setting stage, so that you can work on them, and to ensure your sneaky mind doesn't try to sabotage your progress. But how do you find out? Well, that's the easy part, all you need to do is ask yourself 2 questions...

When you ask yourself these questions, you should take a few moments to *really think about your answers*. You can write your answers down in the boxes provided (or feel free to grab a piece of paper/electronic device to do the same). The first question will help you figure out if there *are* any "secondary gains" that might hinder you in achieving your goal, and the second question will help you to further connect to your goal on a more personal level.

1. "When I reach my goal, will anything be worse?"

I'd like you to imagine that you've already achieved your goal. Connect with that idea fully now. Then think about whether any aspect of your life will have changed for the worse. Think about all possibilities, anything at all; your health, wealth, relationships, ego, emotions, etc. What are you afraid of? If you find that you have an answer for this question, then it may benefit from being addressed (or at least considered) in order to help you move forwards towards your goal.

Take a moment to think about that question now… and feel free to fill in your answer here, if you want to:

When I reach my goal, will anything be worse?"

2. "What will be better once I've reached my goal?"

Again, imagine you've reached your goal successfully, and again, think as broadly as possible when answering this question. What has changed for the *better*, having now achieved your goal? Think about your health, wealth, relationships, ego, emotions, etc. and consider where reaching your goal will have benefited you. Think about how you'll feel about yourself, what will you be thinking, will you be able to do things you haven't been able to do before...

Take a moment to answer that question now...

What will be better once I've reached my goal?

These benefits that you have realised for yourself (assuming you answered the question), will serve to strengthen your will power, to connect you personally to your goal so that you can know you will achieve It, and you *will* know when you *have* achieved it. These benefits will inspire you to give it your all, because you want to succeed at reaching your goal, you will reap the rewards, and you can learn to love being self-motivated by focusing on just how good that is going to feel... #FeelsGoodMan

A final point on goals

You now know how to set yourself effective goals, SMART goals, long and short-term goals, also how to check that your goal works for you, *and* how to motivate yourself towards achieving your goal. A good thing to remember is that your goals don't have to be about how much weight you want to lose! They could be about making changes to your lifestyle, your relationships, your time management, your willpower, anything! You can use these goal techniques to help you improve almost any aspect of your life, just make sure you follow all of the steps mentioned, and you'll be well on your way to improving whatever it is that you wish to improve! #You'reWelcome

Positive Focus
It's important, when making changes in your life, to keep your focus positive, rather than negative. What I mean is, you need to work on moving towards things that you want (your goals), instead of focusing on moving away from what you don't want (such as being fat, not exercising or eating too much). Focusing on avoiding what you *don't* want is kind of like going for a drive in the car, looking at every road sign you come to, and going the opposite direction to all the places that you *don't want to go to*, and hoping that by doing that, you'll end up at your desired destination. Unless you're particularly lucky, it's unlikely you'll reach your goal in this way.

Sure, it's all well and good that you want to stop doing those negative things, but by actively focusing on *not doing them*, you "give them power", which means it's likely you're making it harder for yourself.

If you keep thinking "I won't eat that cake in the cupboard" over and over, the main focal point of that thought is about eating the cake in the cupboard. By focusing, instead, on what you *do* want, such as; "I'm going to fast until 2pm today", then you'll still be achieving the "won't eat that cake" thing, but without needing to think about it directly. Taking away any negative focus and replacing it with something more positive to focus upon will often make your life a lot easier. Do keep positive focus in mind, both when setting your goals, and even when "talking to yourself".

Self-talk
We all talk to ourselves about ourselves, but sometimes we aren't quite as kind (or helpful) as we could be. You've probably heard of "affirmations", the idea that by telling yourself something positive over and over, it will help you to begin believing it, acting upon it, and helping you to become better and better. This is a proven psychological trick that can work great, unfortunately however, it also works equally well in reverse. We are often guilty of giving ourselves "negative affirmations" or telling ourselves over and over why we are no good, or can't do something, or are undeserving of success, and often we don't consciously realise that we're doing it. This means that by telling yourself that you suck, you'll soon start to believe it, and that definitely won't help your progress (or your overall wellbeing and ego). If you notice yourself having negative thoughts, or

thoughts about being unworthy or undeserving of reaching your fasting and health-related goals, mindfulness (again) is the way forwards. A principle of mindfulness is to acknowledge your thoughts and to understand that they are *just* thoughts. So, what I'd like you to do is think of a negative thought of your own, and it can be any thought where you're talking down to yourself. Here are some random examples:

"I don't deserve to lose weight"

"I'm fat and gross"

"I never do anything right"

You get the idea. So, once you've got a thought similar to one of the examples above, specific to you, then I'd like you to take a moment to focus on that thought, to experience how crap it makes you feel when you fuse with it. Once you've done that, then I want you to clear your mind for a moment. Now, take that thought and attach this phrase in front of it; "I'm having the thought that…" and say the thought to yourself again, for example; "I'm having the thought that I don't deserve to lose weight". Try that now with your thought; "I'm having the thought that…"

Isn't it interesting how much less emotional impact there is with the prefixed/reframed thought, in comparison to the original thought? Just by adding 5 words to the start of your negative thought, it becomes much less bothersome. Much flatter. Once you've done that, you can take it a step further with; "I notice that…" so; "I notice that…I'm having the thought that…I don't deserve to lose weight"

What you're doing here is taking yourself away (dissociating) from your thought, so that you can simply acknowledge it, without letting it affect you. This is a highly useful strategy, because you've got to remember that *thoughts are just thoughts*…they're not facts. Thoughts are made up from information in your head. Some thoughts are less true than others. It will help you to become aware that your thoughts are just thoughts, and you can do this as you notice that you're having the thought that your thoughts are just thoughts. #ThoughtInception

A final point on self-talk is that, as well as speaking positively to yourself about yourself, it's also important to speak positively to yourself about your decisions and choices. Let's go back to the cake in the cupboard example from before; we already know you're not going to have the cake until after you finish fasting, but the way that you tell yourself you're not going to have it can make the not-having-it process either easier or harder. Here are two very similar "thoughts" you could have about the cake, notice which one seems more helpful, and which is less:

"I can't have the cake until I stop fasting"

"I won't have the cake until I stop fasting"

The "can't" thought is less helpful, this is because you are imposing a limitation upon yourself, as if you are being *made* to not have the cake. Basically, you are telling yourself that you are being deprived of cake. Whereas, with the "won't" thought, *you* are the one who is in control. You are choosing not to have the cake until you allow yourself to. Both thoughts are aiming towards the exact same outcome (no cake), but how much easier will it be to accomplish, knowing that you are in control? If you notice a thought is causing you some internal conflict, then challenge it and change it to a different thought, a more positive-focused thought. Give yourself control with the way that you talk to yourself, rather than setting limitations for yourself.

Know you're worth it
Sometimes, we can forget how important we are. No, I don't mean in a narcissistic "I'm the best, bow down before me and worship!" kinda way. I mean, we are important to ourselves, and we are important to others (though we might not always feel it or connect to our own innate importance). Think about people that rely on you, those who care for you, those who've enjoyed being with you, whether family, friends or colleagues. You *are* important to others, but you've got to remember to be important

to yourself too. You've got to give a shit about you, because sometimes we're all too busy to put other people first, which means sometimes it might *seem* like no one else cares (because they're busy too), so, make sure *you* care about yourself. Treat yourself like you'd treat someone you love; speak positively to and about yourself, compliment yourself, give yourself a break when the going gets tough, and know that you're worth it.

Some people never give themselves a chance, and always stand in their own way. Some people feel undeserving of success, or that they don't have the right to enjoy their lives, and do things that *they* want to do… Well, I'm here to tell you that if you're one of those people, you can put a sock in it. You are human, like me, like everyone else reading this book. We all have the equal right to be happy, to be healthy and to enjoy life, regardless of what anyone or anything may have told you in the past! You know now that your beliefs can be challenged and changed, and not just your beliefs about food, but your beliefs about *you*. So, challenge your beliefs that are holding you back. Get out of your own way and you will learn to accept the fact that you deserve what we all deserve… and perhaps you deserve even more than the rest of us, in back payment! Because you do deserve a chance. You wouldn't want to make somebody that you care for feel unworthy and undeserving, would you? You'd want that person, the person you love, to be able to enjoy their lives as much as possible, wouldn't you? Yes…

So, learn to love yourself…

…because you're fucking worth it.

Make it about more than just you
Perhaps it might be a tricky concept, putting yourself first, before your friends and family, but it doesn't have to *just* be about you. If you're concerned about caring for yourself too much, or even worried about appearing self-obsessed or self-centred, you can find a way to make your fasting process include those that care for you too, albeit indirectly. Remind yourself that you're doing it for them as well as you, losing weight so that you will be healthier, so that you will be able to see your children grow up, or spend time with your parents, or enjoy spending time with friends, doing different things that you might not have been able to do so well when you were bigger. If you're highly focused on (and motivated by) those you care for, then thinking about your fasting process in a way that includes them can help you to engage with it even more fully and in a way that is congruent with you.

Expectation vs intention
These two concepts may seem similar but, though both are useful, they are, in fact, very different. Lots of literature tells us that we should go into things

with the "expectation" that we will succeed, upholding a strong belief that things will just go your way ...and that's fine, that's positive, but it's not enough. Expectation is very external, meaning it is reliant on forces outside of yourself, and things that are beyond your control. "Intention" is different and *is* within your control. Intention takes expectation and gives it a huge boost, by factoring in yourself as an influencing factor. Who could better influence the outcome of a situation in your life than you? If you simply "expect" to get a job and you go to the interview having done no prep, and you turn up looking like you just rolled out of bed, is it likely that "the universe will provide"? No, why would it? So, do not just "expect" that things will go your way. Make them go your way by "intending" for it to happen. Look at what you want to achieve, set your goals and targets, and work towards them with a strong intention. Aim to meet your purpose with laser-focus, with this burning intention and desire always at the forefront of the decisions you make and the reactions you choose to have.
#IntentionExceedsExpectations

Willpower
Willpower can be thought of as your response to an "internal conflict". The American Psychological Association defines willpower as; "The ability to delay gratification, resisting short-term temptations in order to meet long-term goals, and the capacity to override an unwanted thought, feeling or impulse".

Everyone has willpower, and each person's willpower may vary. Willpower varies both "globally" (i.e. across the board, in every aspect of your life, as influenced by your mood, and other factors at the time), and also it can vary depending on which aspect of your life you're applying it to. For example; someone may have strong willpower relating to eating healthy foods, yet poor control over trying to quit smoking cigarettes, or poor willpower relating to *not* speaking their mind (and getting themselves into trouble), but strong enough willpower to manage to haul their ass to the gym at 6am every day.

We all have the ability to use our willpower (if we choose to), but we *also* have the ability to develop the *strength* of our willpower beyond where it currently stands. Willpower is like a muscle, and like a muscle you can strengthen it with use. We all have different sized muscles and are able to exercise our muscles at different intensities for different periods of time, but it's also true that *anybody* can develop their muscles if they truly intend to. Also, it's worth noting at the start of this section that, the same as with building muscles, if you try and exercise your willpower muscle *too much*, it can become tired and (temporarily) weaken, meaning it needs time for recovery. So, it's good to build in "rest periods" for your willpower, rather than trying to exercise it 24/7 in every aspect of your life, and having it become burnt out. Luckily, the fasting plans presented in this book are designed to work well with this exact principle, automatically allowing you to "recharge" your willpower in between fasts.

There are various different ways in which you can develop and improve your willpower, but it's important that you don't try and do too much too soon, because this may require more willpower than you currently have available, or more than you're comfortable using. For instance, I've said previously that you *could* do 20-hour fasts instead of 18-hour fasts, and that it may help you to lose weight faster, but if you've not gotten used to the 18-hour ones yet, then the 20-hour ones are going to take a bit more willpower and might be harder to complete. So, make sure when you're on the route to developing your fasting/fat loss willpower, that you do it in "baby steps". For instance, if, after finishing the book, you decide to cut down on eating unhealthy foods, then you'll probably do better by eliminating them gradually, rather than taking everything away all at once. Sure, it would be healthier to substitute a whole shopping basket full of crap with a whole basket full of fruit and veg, but your willpower may not quite be ready for that yet. However, if you swapped just a quarter of the basket out for healthier stuff, it becomes much more achievable, and less of a jump.

The great thing about willpower is, each time you successfully use it, it becomes stronger. Each time you exercise your willpower you'll need to think about it less, because when you begin using your willpower effectively, it will become a habit. It'll become something that you just do. But the opposite is also true, meaning each time you try and use willpower and fail, or you say "fuck it" too often, your willpower will likely reduce/stay the same. Luckily, the odd slip up isn't a big deal, but you need to ensure that you make what you're doing achievable, as this will help you to successfully use your willpower as often as possible. Repetition is the way that we build habits, so ensure that the willpower-habit you're building and repeating is a positive one. You won't build masses of willpower *all in one go*, but with constant repetition, it *will* happen. It's kind of like the age-old question; "how do you eat an elephant?" ...well, one bite at a time of course! #TheElephantIsAMetaphorForYourWillpower #DontEatTheElephants #DumboBurger

Willpower improvement strategies
So how can you actively work on your willpower, outside of the fasting process? You have plenty of options, and if you can commit to doing a couple of these a day, then you'll be well on the way to improving your willpower, so it's ready to use in a pinch.

Note: In order to benefit from these strategies, again, you have to actually do them, not just read and forget about them!

Most of these things are relatively simple concepts, such as actively working to sit up straight, instead of slouching (if you slouch). Leave yourself a note where you sit, reminding you to sit up straight. Each time you notice it (and if you're not still sitting up), use your willpower to do so for as long as you can. This simple act will help to improve your willpower globally, not just in relation to sitting up straight. Initially, you might notice that it's not comfortable, and that it takes some actual effort. This is true, but the more you do it, the easier it will become, and not only will you be forming the habit of using your willpower, but you will also be forming the positive habit of sitting up straight.

You can set yourself time-based tasks, such as brushing your teeth mindfully for two minutes (paying attention to only brushing your teeth and focusing on no other thoughts or distractions). How about doing a monotonous activity for as long as you can, such as clicking a pen, or squeezing a ball, these work well because as well as the time element, your muscles will start to ache too, so it's a real test of willpower and "mind over matter". Perhaps you could challenge yourself to use your non-dominant hand for a set period of time for whatever it is that you're doing (maybe not during your job, if you need to write stuff/use your hand for precision purposes). This works because you have to consciously think about what you're doing, and your coordination won't be as good with your non-dominant hand.

Prefer a less physical way to improve willpower? Look no further than your mouth. Work on correcting your speech, and speaking as properly as you can, in any-and-all situations. Work on using full words rather than shortened ones (hi/hello, 'sup/what's up, mmm/yes), work on cutting out "ums" and "errs", have a go at reducing your swearing (#FuckThat), etc. Again, this will take effort, and you don't have to make *all* of the changes I just suggested, so long as you actively change the way you speak in some way (ideally for the better), and in a way that you have to actively think about.

Active distraction is a great way to support the willpower-strengthening process, so rather than just doing nothing when you're facing a test of willpower, and thinking; "no, I'm not going to eat", it can be more useful to do something completely different, to distract yourself from the very thought. It can be as simple as thinking something else... Think about an upcoming event, or a past positive experience. Perhaps try and remember all the lyrics to a song, or even visualise yourself in a year or two from now, do anything to interrupt your thought process, in a way that keeps you engaged for a minute or two. If there's a food in front of you on your journey, or if you're standing talking to someone and there's food in your eyeline, reposition yourself so that it isn't. You can do many random things in order to distract yourself from what you're thinking about, such as doing a little dance (if you're in public you may be too embarrassed to carry on thinking about anything else …or if you're good, you might even get some tips, lol). Perhaps try and think of as many words you can that rhyme with "night". Maybe you could set a stopwatch on your phone and see if you can accurately count the seconds up to a minute without looking at it… the possibilities for distracting yourself are endless.

As well as distracting yourself from the thing you want to do, you can also simply postpone it until later. Say there's a cupcake in the cupboard, and you want to eat it. Let yourself know that you *can* have it, but only after you get back from walking the dog, or reading 30 pages of a novel, or whatever. Delaying an immediate, knee-jerk action still counts as using your willpower, even if you do still do the thing later on in the day (or another day).

Some of us, however, are better at using this strategy than others, as was demonstrated by the "Stanford Marshmallow Experiment" that was used to test the willpower (or "delayed gratification") of children. Each child was left in a room with a marshmallow, and if he/she managed to resist the marshmallow for the duration of the test (only like 15 minutes or so), then they'd get a second marshmallow as a prize, and could have both. If they ate it during the test, they'd only get the one. Some of the children simply could not resist…

It actually turned out (in the original experiment) that the children who *were* able to wait longer in order to get the larger reward, tended to have better life-outcomes generally. This test also confirmed that scientists are dicks, lol. #LikeGivingCandyToABaby

Relating to fasting, food diaries can be great in order to help you build your willpower (as writing down everything you eat can take a bit of conscious effort), and we've already covered diaries in the previous section. Another tip is to make sure you're not tempting yourself and challenging your willpower unnecessarily. Don't put yourself in situations that make your life difficult. Don't buy crap food that you don't need/want, and if you do have to buy it for other members of the family, have them hide it somewhere that you're not aware of (obviously don't give a 4-year-old the chocolates to hide... that won't end well). Contrary to that last bit of information, you could try doing exactly the opposite and actively carrying something tempting around with you, to prove to yourself that you *can* resist it, even when it's available at any time. Different approaches work for different people, so experiment and find the approach(es) that work best for you.

Connect to past resources

Just for a moment, I'd like you to think about some times when you've used your willpower effectively. Times when you've done things that were challenging, but you did them anyway. Think about times that you stuck to things where other people may have not managed to do what you did, such as; studying, exams, routines, jobs, parenting, eating, exercise, other lifestyle choices, etc. Think back to when you were determined, when you "stuck to it", and just how much willpower and self-control you exercised. Think about how good you felt for not quitting, for pushing through and sticking to your guns. Because you have used your willpower effectively in the past, means you can channel your internal resources for further use in the future.

There's a technique known as "state anchoring" that can take your pre-existing resources and put them "on tap", to use whenever you like. Anchoring is used frequently in hypnotherapy to "anchor" (connect) a positive resource state to a specific physical action (i.e. pressing your fingers together to feel confident). This method is tried & tested, used by sports people, by those engaging in public speaking, by actors, by people looking to improve their lives (to mention just a few), and it works really well. So, if you find yourself struggling or in need of a boost, an anchor will work great! Read through the instructions in full before you do this.

What you'll need to do, as discussed a couple of paragraphs ago, is think back to a time in your life when you had strong willpower, were successful, confident, resourceful (or whatever positive/ resourceful "state of mind" it is that you want to anchor). Then, you'll close your eyes for a while and just remember everything you can about that situation. You can then intensify the feelings and emotions, using your imagination to make the experience as vivid or powerful as you possibly can. Once you're sure the positive feeling/state is at the highest possible peak, then (and only then) you can set your "anchor".

The anchor itself is simply a physical action, and a great anchor for most people is to squeeze the thumb of your right hand to the ring finger/pinkie finger of your right hand... This is an action that we barely ever do, which means you have to actually think about it to do it (as opposed to just touching your thumb and index finger/middle finger together, which happens naturally more often). It works best if it's an action you don't do very often (or at all), because the whole point is that it's a "conscious choice" to experience the anchored feelings, and if you're just touching those fingers together all the time, it'll desensitise your anchor, and won't work.

So, you'll think about your positive experience, build up the intensity of the positive emotions, and then you'll set your anchor at the most intense point by

squeezing your thumb and your finger together...
Once you've done that, release the fingers and forget
about that memory/experience. Take a few
moments to clear your head, and then do it again,
but with a different positive memory/experience,
and repeat the process over and over at least 5 times
(but the more the better). And if you can't remember
any times where you had that "resourceful state"
you're looking for, then just imagine what it *would*
be like (...it's better though, if you can use some real-
life memories). You may be surprised at just how
effective this "mind trick" can be at making you feel
good!

A final point on anchoring. Once you've got your
anchor all set up, if you naturally find yourself in a
positive state; let's say you just made it out of a
birthday party, and you didn't have any cake because
you were fasting. When you leave the party, and you
feel that sense of accomplishment like "oh yeah, I
have great willpower. I didn't eat that cake!", it's at
that point where you can use your anchor again,
which will add the feelings from this actual, present
positive experience into your anchor. Just focus on
the feeling as you're feeling it, build it up, really feel
it, and squeeze those fingers together again! The
more times you "recharge" your anchor like this, the
more effective it's going to be!

A willpower lifestyle

So, we've covered a whole bunch of things you can do in order to build your willpower, but you've got to remember that your lifestyle can have a massive impact on willpower too. Sleep, again, is one of these things. Sleep reduces stress and improves how our brain works, so not only does having a good night's sleep help us to lose weight more effectively, but it also improves our willpower (a coincidence? Maybe, maybe not). Appropriate exercise and good nutrition can also help to develop the right kind of environment required for strong willpower and are therefore important. You'll learn more about those in the next chapters, along with a bit of information about alcohol. Alcohol, as we know, decreases willpower. So, if you drink a lot, you may be making life harder for yourself. Just something to consider.

Stress is a big one and can have a massive impact on your life in many different ways, especially your health. When we are stressed our bodies produce cortisol (amongst other things), which can cause increased blood pressure, lower sex drive, reduced immune system, it can even supress the digestive system (which can cause weight issues), and guess what... it can reduce your willpower! Argh!

Stress is a natural part of life. It's tied in with our "fight or flight" response, a process that is designed to keep us safe. However, we are not supposed to be in a *constant* state of fight or flight. Pressures of modern life are much different to anything we would have ever experienced during the hunter-gatherer part of our evolutionary existence. Stress is supposed to save us from attack, to give us energy to run or fight, not to seethe about Mary at the office not pulling her weight, or the kids answering you back at home... So, the challenges of modern life can chronically trigger our stress response, meaning the production of cortisol is much more frequent and long lasting. You do not want this.

Again, diet and exercise help with stress. Less alcohol, caffeine, nicotine (and other stimulants) can help to reduce stress too. A great way to really nip stress in the bud though, is with both mindfulness (which we've spoken about already) and meditation. Daily meditation (or daily self-hypnosis) can be very useful to incorporate into your lifestyle, whether to combat stress or as a "pre-emptive strike", managing stress before you're even stressed. You don't have to be a hippy, or a middle-aged woman who wears lots of purple beads in order to meditate, in fact it can be really beneficial for almost anyone. I also mentioned self-hypnosis. Self-hypnosis and meditation seem very similar on the face of it, but are not quite the same. Meditation is more about clearing the mind, whereas self-hypnosis is more about focusing intensely on an idea/goal, however, both are very relaxing, and can help you to increase willpower. They do this by getting you to pay attention to your thoughts, by building your own self-awareness, by increasing your ability to focus, and by reducing your stress. When you engage in meditation, you're going to want to aim for at least 10 minutes per day, to get the most benefit from it. 10 minutes is less than 1% of your day, so it's definitely an achievable amount of time to invest. Though it might seem like an alien concept, especially if you've never done anything like it before, the stress-reduction benefits alone make it worthwhile. A great starting point for learning how to meditate is Wikihow.com, where their article walks you through all the steps of meditation and how to get the most from it.

Wikihow.com also has a walk-through for self-hypnosis, however, it can be better to visit a hypnotherapist in person in order to set up the self-hypnosis process more effectively, as it's a bit more in-depth than meditation, and can help if you have experience going into hypnosis beforehand. Unlike meditation, during self-hypnosis, it's useful to give yourself simple "suggestions" (kind of like "affirmations") relating to your goal, such as; "if I notice myself feeling stressed, I will take 3 deep breaths, and relax" or even more simply; "I am feeling more relaxed than ever before, able to take anything in my stride". Obviously, these suggestions are simple and easy to understand, but they need to be, as if you give yourself too much to remember, you'll forget, and that might stress you out (lol). Like I said, self-hypnosis is often best set up with a hypnotherapist after a full hypnotherapy session relating to your own personal goals. By doing it this way, it will be most effective (just ensure that your hypnotherapist is comfortable teaching self-hypnosis before you book a session, as some don't do it, so shop around).

Outside of self-hypnosis and meditation, you can still use your mind to deal with stress. As mentioned before, taking deep breaths can help you to reduce stress, this is a scientific fact. Long exhalation (breathing out) activates the parasympathetic nervous system, or your "relaxation response", so it can be good practice, when stressed, to exhale for a longer amount of time than your inhale. So, just breathe normally for a moment now... breathing in and out for the same amount of time for both your inhale and exhale. Notice how nothing really changes... Now breathe in, but when you breathe out, extend the breath, make it longer. Do this a couple of times now; normal breath in, longer breath out, and now, notice how much more relaxed you feel...

Note: This also works in reverse (but I don't recommend trying it). By extending the inhale and shortening the exhale, you would become more stressed and on-edge, as this is your "sympathetic" nervous system responding, preparing you for fight/flight, which is why you may GASP if something noisy/scary happens around you.

Finally, on the topic of stress, simple visualisations (or using your imagination) can also help you to relax. Think about something in your life now that's stressing you out; work, partner, school, kids, friends, family, whatever makes you feel stressed at this very moment. Get a sense of that stress now. Really connect to it… (and I wonder if your breathing changes, lol) …and now, *in a moment*, I want you to close your eyes and imagine you are in the most relaxing place on earth, with only the people you want, doing whatever you like. It can be any place, real or imagined, but the perfect setting for you to be 100% relaxed. And if you're not a particularly "visual person", know that you can simply close your eyes and imagine what it *would be like* to imagine that scene… that wonderful relaxing place. You can just get a sense of what it would be like to be there, in your own way, the perfect setting for you to be 100% relaxed, as you take a moment to do that, and go to that place as you close your eyes now…

So, having done that, notice how different you feel. Having begun the exercise feeling stressed, and then by simply focusing on a super-relaxing scene, perhaps you may have found that you're more relaxed than you were before (if you fully engaged in using your imagination). Our imagination is powerful, we can imagine ourselves sick, we can imagine ourselves better, we can use our imagination to help us win, to succeed, to overcome. Trust that your imagination can help you, even when *part of you* is stressing out. Know that you have this within you, a part of your mind that can easily shut down that stress, that can stamp out that fire, like a wild rhino would stamp out a fire to save the bush around it... You have control over the rhino of your mind. So, use it. #WhatsWithAllTheAfricaReferencesAnyway #AwhimawayAwhimaway

Life is a rollercoaster ride
During fasting, as with anything, you've gotta expect ups and downs, and whether it's fluctuations in motivation or in weight, these ups and downs are normal and to be expected. You wouldn't start a new job and expect every day to be awesome, because of course there are gonna be days where you feel less-good. Life can be chaotic and often unpredictable, but if you're having a hard time of it, it can be worth thinking back to positive times where you *were* coping well, or where you *were* experiencing success (we've all had them, in one form or another), and simply take a moment to imagine yourself back at that time, connecting fully to the memory. By doing this, you'll often be able to change your mood from negative, to positive in the blink of an eye. It's similar to how smiling can combat a bad mood... If you smile, even when you're not feeling particularly happy, your mood will lighten as your brain releases dopamine, serotonin and other feel-good chemicals, and you'll feel a bit (or a lot) better. By accessing and engaging with past positive memories, the same kind of thing happens, and especially if the past positive

memory was a *really* good one, it'll generally help you to push through your current emotional state and get back on track. It's useful to pre-prepare a couple of positive memories for this purpose, so that they come to mind more easily, as when you're in a low mood, positive memories can seem harder to come by.

As I mentioned a moment ago, sometimes we get fluctuations in weight, and sometimes you might find your fat-loss progress slows down or "plateaus", which can be caused by various different factors. It's worth remembering that a plateau is not the end of the world, and if your progress *were* to plateau, you've just got to keep doing what you're doing. Think of a plateau kind of like a speed bump in the road... So, you might go up a bit, but if you keep going in the right direction, you'll go back down. This tiny little speed bump isn't a good enough reason to stop your journey completely, it's not going to make you turn around. Sure, it might shake you up a bit as you drive over it, but eventually, it will be in the rear-view mirror, a thing of the past, and you'll just carry on driving, pedal to the metal, further and further down the road to success, until you reach your goal. #TryNotToGetASpeedingTicket

Remember why you started
You're reading this book for a reason, make sure you keep this reason in mind as you go onwards. Hell, write the reason(s) that you're fasting inside the

front cover of the book to remind you why you started, so if you ever pick up the book again for additional motivation, or for a refresher, it's right there on the first page. The reason you started fasting in the first place is the best piece of motivation you can give to your future self. It sounds simple now, but in 2, 6, 12, 24 months, that simple piece of information may very well be inspiring enough to kick your ass back into gear and bust you through any plateaus that you might be facing!

Embrace the discipline
Long-term, sustainable weight loss can take work, just like many things that are worth doing, there aren't always "quick fixes" available, sometimes it takes good old-fashioned dedication and self-discipline in order to meet our goals. Discipline isn't something that needs to be endured, in fact it's something that can actually be *enjoyed*. Take pleasure in your ability to stick firmly to your guns, because then, even if everything around you were going to shit, you'll know that what you're doing is a constant, it's reliable, it's a part of the new you. So, if you're hungry, accept it and allow yourself to feel it. Make yourself experience it fully, connect to it, get to know it, explore exactly how it feels, and embrace it, because this "hunger" is the feeling of success. It's a feeling that can remind you that if you can do this, then you can do just about anything!

Soon, you will learn to enjoy sticking to this plan and pushing yourself in the right direction, and by relying on your own self-discipline, you'll do something that you can be proud to have achieved, because if you give it your all, you *will* be proud of yourself when you reach (or even surpass) your goals. When you choose to embrace the discipline required to stick with this plan for the long-run, soon you'll be looking in the mirror, not only seeing a leaner, healthier version of yourself, but also a determined, strong-willed person, a new version of you that has the ability to exercise self-discipline in order to get whatever it is that you want. So, embrace the discipline, harness it, and use it to succeed!

Download your Hypno-Fasting MP3

So, you've read through the section on programming your mind for success, and now you understand that there are many ways to make your fasting and fat-loss process more effective... You can now take this knowledge and understanding to the next level, by listening to the hypnosis MP3 that comes included with this book. The MP3 has been specifically designed to complement the **Hypno-Fasting** process and to aid and support you in your fat-loss journey.

Download your hypnosis MP3 (for free) by visiting: **hypno-fasting.com/mp3**

Once there, enter the password: **TIME2GETFASTING**

(...and remember it's case-sensitive, so all in capital letters ...except the "2", obviously! lol)

Once you've accessed the page, simply enter your email address, and you'll then receive an email with a download link, so that you can download a copy of the MP3 onto *any device* that you wish.

If, before listening to the MP3, you have any questions or concerns about *hypnosis*, check out the FAQs section on the MP3 download page itself, or in the download email. That said, if you can wait, do feel free to bookmark this page and listen to the MP3 a bit later, because the book's not *quite* done yet...

How to Eat Healthier

OK, so we're finished talking about the actual process of fasting, and we've gone through a whole load of tips and tactics to help you succeed as easily and effortlessly as possible. You could stop reading at this point, and just go and do it... Or you can keep reading and learn how to make your results happen *even faster* by using the food that you eat more effectively. You may find that just by refreshing your knowledge or learning to look at food from a slightly different perspective, that you can make some small but high-impact changes. Don't worry though, I'm gonna stay true to the rest of the book and keep this section super simple too, just 'cause I know you love it!

Disclaimer: I am not a qualified dietician. I'm not even an un-qualified dietician, so although the information contained here is correct to the best of my knowledge and personal experience, don't take it as scientific fact. Some of the calorie information may not be 100% accurate, but it should be pretty darn close. Also, nutritional plans work differently for different people, so again, it may behove you to do some research to corroborate what I'm saying before you make any dietary changes.

FYI during this section, if I mention that you *can't* or *shouldn't* have something during your fast, it basically just means it contains calories, so if you're doing a true fast (i.e. the "Full-Timer Plan") then you're not gonna want to put any calories into your body. If, however, you're on one of the calorie restriction fasts, then obviously you *can* have whatever it is, but it *will* count towards your daily calories.

Fancy a drink?

Let's start off light and talk about drinks. Drinking is very important, but people often make the mistake of not counting their drinks towards their daily calorie intake. Unfortunately, pretty much any drink (other than water) will contain calories, and if it doesn't, it'll probably contain a truck-load of questionable chemicals to make it taste like it does. So, as a committed faster, you must always remember that drinks can make you fat too, I mean, why do you think they call it a "beer belly"? I rest my case. Anyway, here's a brief overview of the kind of liquids you should and shouldn't guzzle down your throat hole... #NotThatKindOfLiquid #DirtyMind

Note: "Man-juice" has calories too! Apparently about 5-7 calories per teaspoonful! So please, if you're fasting, lay off the blowjobs... Just one "portion" (*ahem*) probably wouldn't be too detrimental, but if you're at a college party playing the "soggy biscuit" game, well, the same cannot be said.

*(If you have no idea what soggy biscuit is, please **do not ever** search UrbanDictionary.com for details, lol)*

Water

As I have already mentioned a couple of times throughout the book; water is your friend. If you are able to be so disciplined and awesome that the only thing you drink is water, then you're already gonna be off to a great start. Water has no calories, it will flush your system, it energises your muscles, keeps your skin looking good, it helps your kidneys more effectively get rid of all the crap in your body, and it helps ease constipation, and all that shit. #PooPuns

Water is the best way to rehydrate, it is absorbed into your body fast, and quickly begins to work its voodoo magic! Water can stave off muscle cramps, fight hangovers and headaches, stop you feeling so tired, and the list goes on... Now that's what I call high quality H^2O!

Also, when it comes to helping you with your fast, water is the King of the beverages! Drink it whilst fasting to ensure you won't feel hungry. Drink it before (and during) your meals, and you'll get full-up faster than if you were just eating food by itself, meaning you'll eat less, have less calories to burn off, and end up being so goddamn sexy you'll wanna rip your own clothes off every time you walk past even the most mildly reflective surface.

So, unless you're literally drowning, I think you'll agree that water is just awesome. Make water your go-to drink of choice. About 2 litres of water a day is the generally accepted recommendation, but you may want to drink a bit more if you are exercising, or if you have a physically demanding occupation/hobby. Oh, and by the way, if you're not used to drinking very much, get used to peeing. Lots and lots of peeing.

Warning: Yes, drinking lots of water is good, but don't drink too much water, because you could actually die. Like, literally. If you're drinking around 2-4 litres of water a day, that should be fine (depending on your body weight), but when you drink 5+ litres you could be getting into risky territory. "Water intoxication" occurs when you drink so much water in a relatively short period of time that your blood becomes diluted, this can lead to complications and even death. Apparently, it takes around 6 litres of water to kill a 165lb person... So yeah, keep that fact in mind, and go easy on the sky juice!

Hot Drinks
Don't drop it like it's hot, because hot drinks can work really well alongside your fasting plan. I said it before, but it's worth repeating that you can pretty much drink as many cups of tea or coffee as you like ...but there is a catch; as soon as you add milk, cream, sugar, honey (or whatever else you would add to your hot drink to make it taste less like the original drink itself), then you're adding calories to the drink. This means you won't be able to have it during your fast.

Also, it should go without saying that Hot Chocolates, Cappuccinos, Pumpkin Spiced Lattes (could you be any more of a white girl stereotype?) and all those kinds of drinks are out. They all contain calories. In fact, some of those choices contain a *lot* of calories. Here's a list of some common hot drinks and their calorie contents (per cup), just to give you an idea:

Black coffee	**<2 calories**
Black tea	**<2 calories**
Tea w/milk & 2 sugars	**40 calories**
Café latte	**99 calories**
Cappuccino	**120 calories**
Store bought hot chocolate	**230 calories**
Pumpkin Spice Latte w/cream	**410 calories (fuck!)**

Note: The symbol < means "less than", in case you failed high-school mathematics.

As you can see, plain black tea and black coffee are under 2 calories (which, for all intents and purposes, means 0 calories), so drinking them plain means you can pretty much have your fill. So, don't panic, you can still get your caffeine kick in the morning! Coffee is a great stimulant, and it's said that caffeine can actually help you to lose fat, it's also thermogenic (increases body heat), and you quite frequently find caffeine in these otherwise-questionable "fat burning" supplements that have become popular recently.

Obviously, caffeine can disrupt your sleep patterns to some extent (not to mention making you super twitchy after, like, 4 cups), so if you're not used to it, you might wanna start off slowly. If you are sensitive to caffeine but love the taste of coffee, there are loads of caffeine-free coffees on the market which, if you get a good one, taste pretty much just the same as regular coffee (but without the buzz). Decent caffeine-free tea can be a little harder to come by, but if you search for "Red Bush" or "Rooibos" tea, that's another caffeine-free alternative to normal tea.

Another great tea alternative is green tea (which *does* contain caffeine). Benefits of green tea supposedly include a slight increase in metabolic rate, appetite reduction, fat burning properties, improved brain function, it's high in antioxidants (which may lower risk of cancer) and it's said that green tea promotes a reduced risk of other diseases and diabetes too. The benefits of drinking green tea are apparently so good, that they may even outweigh the fact that it tastes like Satan's asshole. Seriously, it's horrendous. Also, some of the benefits (especially the antioxidants) would be lost if consumed with milk, so you've got no choice but to "enjoy" the flavor of the tea on its own. That said, if you do want the benefits of green tea, you should always go for the tea itself and not for "green tea supplements", which are apparently much less effective (or so I hear). To reap the full rewards of green tea, you're meant to drink at least 4 cups per day, so, Bon Appétit! #RatherYouThanMe

I personally (during my pre-fasting-era) used to drink tea with at least two sugars and about 25% of my mug would be filled with milk. I started fasting and decided that I actually wasn't a huge fan of tea with no milk/sugar, so I decided to try black coffee instead, and I must say; black coffee rocks! Black coffee is now my drink of choice, whether I'm fasting or not (and I'm even on the caffeine-free version now too – much less twitchy). Somehow, I managed to ditch the sugar too, but if you really can't deal with having an un-sweetened hot drink, then luckily for you, you can use sugar-free sweeteners during a fast (because they generally have 0 calories). Again, be aware that these sweeteners are usually pretty unnatural, and may contain all sorts of weird ingredients that your body might not like very much. It's up to you to research whether the stuff that you stick in your body is good for you or not.

Milk
Moo, bitch, get out the whey! Milk is totally delicious, who doesn't love a nice cool, refreshing glass of cow juice? (apart from lactose intolerant folks I guess...) Milk *does* have calories, so unfortunately, it's no good during fast-periods, but otherwise, milk isn't a bad choice of refreshing beverage. Keep an eye on what type of milk you're drinking, however, because not all milks are created

equal. Here are the calories (per cup) contained in the top 3 types of milk available to buy. Oh, and cream too:

Non-fat/Skim Milk	**90 calories**
Reduced-fat/Semi-Skimmed/1-2%	**115 calories**
Whole/full-fat Milk	**150 calories**
Cream	**470 calories**

So, you need to be careful what you're putting in your tea/coffee, you could go from under 10 calories to over 100 with a little pour! Also, I'm not gonna waste your time talking about almond milk, coconut milk, soy milk and all that type of stuff, because if you're the sort of person who drinks it, you probably know what it contains already! (That was pretty tactful, right? #BloodyHippies)

Squash/Fruit Concentrate/Cordial/Powders

As a rule, most concentrates (i.e. a liquid or powder that you add to water to make it taste like something else) will contain some calories, unless stated otherwise on the packaging. Unless it's a 0-calorie version, it's something to avoid whilst on your fast.

Fruit Juice

Orange juice, apple juice, all those drinks are healthy right? Well, I mean, juice isn't as bad as some things, but it's definitely not the same as eating the equivalent piece of fruit. This is because of all the added sugar. An 8oz/200ml glass of OJ (usually) contains around 2.5x more sugar than a good old-fashioned orange (and you get next to none of the healthy fibre you'd get whilst eating the fruit either). Most fruit juices will be 110+ calories per cup, so you can't have fruit juice while fasting. Same goes for those outrageously expensive smoothies all the hipsters are drinking. Ditch 'em.

Carbonated/Fizzy Drinks
Fizzy drinks are basically just bad for you (sorry, your mother was right). I mean, yeah, they can be delicious, sure, but you wouldn't put 7 spoonfuls of sugar in any of your other drinks, and apparently that's how much sugar is in a can of Coke. Whether you're male or female, just one can would put you over your daily recommended sugar allowance (i.e. recommended by doctors). Also, you've got to wonder what fizzy drinks do to your insides if they'll almost completely disintegrate a mouse (seriously, Google "Mountain Dew Mouse Experiment" it's pretty grim – don't watch if you're squeamish). If after watching the mouse video, you still want to drink fizzy drinks, then well done, that's an achievement (either that, or you have no eyes)!

Diet/sugar-free fizzy drinks generally have no calories, which means you *can* have them whilst fasting if you want to. The problem is, diet drinks (artificially sweetened) make your body think it's getting sugar when it isn't, and this is where insulin problems could start (or be worsened). Not to mention the fact that carbonated drinks, whether diet or not, are terrible for your teeth (and probably your insides too, judging by the mouse). But like I said, I'm just here to present some information, and you can make your own decision about what type of shit you put into your body. You're big enough to make your own decisions. ;-)

So yes, you can have sugar free/diet soda during your fast, but no, you can't have the regular, sugar-filled ones. #FirstWorldProblems #DiabetesInACan

Alcohol
If you hadn't already realised, alcohol contains calories (7 calories per gram, in fact), and you can't drink and fast (it's a shame, I know, lol). Anyway, here's a list of the calorie contents of some popular alcoholic beverages:

Beer (Lager)	**180 calories per pint**
Cider	**210 calories per pint**
Red Wine	**125 calories per small glass**
White Wine	**120 calories per small glass**
Spirits	**100 calories per 25ml measure**
JägerBomb	**225 calories**

Generally, we find that people who enjoy alcohol tend to not stop at just a single drink, and when one has had a few drinkies, one generally tends to become more prone to overindulging in other ways, doesn't one?

You don't often hear of people going out to get drunk, and at the end of the night stopping at the salad bar, do you? Being drunk generally goes hand-in-hand with being sloppy and making poor life choices, (whether led by your stomach, your drunk-brain or other "organs" lower down).

Like to binge drink? Well if you are hardcore enough to drink a whole 70cl bottle of whisky in one sitting (more like a laying), then you'd consume a total of around 1,700 calories. If you're a rowdy Englishman up Ye Olde Pube, and you drink 12 fackin' pints of lager, you'd have consumed around 2,100 calories. So, binge drinking and being overweight, well, they often go together …unless you're Lemmy from Motörhead that is. #RIPLemmy

Aside from all of the calories contained in alcohol, some types of alcohol *also* contain estrogen (the primary female sex hormone), which can increase fat storage! So, as fun as alcohol might be, if you're looking to lose fat then it's probably time to put down the bottle and reacquaint yourself with Mr Water …or at least *reduce* your alcohol consumption a bit. But hey, I like a scotch as much as the next guy, so you have to figure out what's more important to you. Do you want abs, or do you want a six pack…of beer? Most people aren't fortunate enough to have both!

OK, let's eat!
So, we've covered drinks, now let's move onto solids. Food is great, but again, not all food is made equal. All food, however, is made up of those three macronutrients that we mentioned before:

- Protein (4 calories per gram)
- Carbs/Carbohydrates (4 calories per gram)
- Fat/Lipids (9 calories per gram)

Now, just by looking at that, you'd assume that I'm going to tell you to ditch foods that are high in fat, right? Well I'm not, because actually, if all we had to eat was natural food (i.e. meat, fruit and vegetables, nuts, eggs, etc.) the thing you'd generally be getting a lot less of (apart from diabetes) would be carbs. Sure, you'd get carbs in potatoes, fruit, and a small amount in vegetables, but not to the same extent as you would by eating chips, fries, pizza, chocolate, ice cream, and all of that processed crap that the food companies want you to buy.

If I were to give you one piece of dietary advice that would probably help you to shift a chunk of weight all by itself, it would be to cut down (or cut out) white carbs and sugary sweet crap. When you eat protein and fat, they generally make you feel fuller, faster. Carbs however, tend to do the opposite, and seem to make us hungrier, and that hunger generally makes us want more carbs (those sneaky bastards!)

Now, I'm not saying cut out *all* carbs, because going on a low-carb diet alongside a fasting plan may be too much for your body to take, and your energy levels may drop significantly (as carbs are a great source of quick-release energy) and having low energy sucks. However, if you simply reduce/remove the *crappy processed carbs* from your diet, you'll be off to a good start. Here are some of the main things you could consider ditching:

- Crisps/potato chips
- Fries
- White potatoes (you could replace with sweet potatoes)
- White breads/buns/bagels (replace with brown/wholegrain versions)
- White rice (replace with brown rice)
- White pasta (replace with… you get the gist)
- Crackers & biscuits
- Breakfast cereals
- Cakes
- Cookies
- Candy
- Chocolate
- Ice cream
- Dried fruit (yup, it's much worse, carb-wise, than normal fruit)

So basically, it could be a good idea to ditch anything that contains sugar or white flour (and if you wanted to make it even more effective, you could completely swear off all types of flour/bread/pasta/rice/sugar etc.). If you must have something floury, then try and make it brown/wholegrain, because it's much better for you.

I did mention the whole fat-not-being-as-bad-as-carbs idea, and though half-right, it can also be half wrong. If you're eating a pack of bacon, a block of cheese and half a stick of butter every day, sure it's low carb, but it's a lot of "bad fat" (and also amounts to way too many calories)! Good fats are "unsaturated fats" or "monounsaturated fats", which can be found in the likes of nuts, fatty fish, flax, olive oil, avocados, seeds, etc. (i.e. natural food that occurs naturally in nature). A cheese-toastie smothered in butter, however, is not naturally occurring. You can't go out hunting in the wilderness expecting to find a deep-fried bacon and cream cheese bagel, lurking in the undergrowth. That kind of food is all man-made, processed, and it's a bad combination of macronutrients...

The combination of doom
By creating all of these delicious types of unnatural food, we have created something that doesn't generally occur in nature, and that is a "ratio". This ratio is an equal (or fairly close) amount of carbs and fat in one food item.

If you think about pretty much all types of natural food, they generally contain either:

- Just carbs
- Mostly protein, but with some fat
- Mostly fat, but with some protein
- Protein, fat and a tiny amount of carbs

Look at most types of junk food, and what they generally contain:

- Lots of carbs and lots of fat together

Sure, some of the things (like sweets/candies) are pure sugar and no fat, but at the same time, that is not natural sugar, if it was, you'd be eating a piece of fruit/honey. The real problems are the carb/fat combos, the pizzas, burgers, fries, cakes, donuts, bagels, chocolate and deep-fried-anythings... These things are addictive, and they're not something we're naturally accustomed to dealing with. Now, obviously pretty much all "junk food" fits into this category, so you *could* do yourself a huge favour by ditching the terrible junk that modern society has tricked you into cramming into your food-hole, and instead go for foods that are more natural/healthy. Your fat will thank you for it (by buggering off).

Pay attention to what you're eating
Pretty simple idea, right? Paying attention to what you're eating. Well, it's sometimes not quite as easy as that. For one thing, some of us get into a dire state known as a "food trance". This is where you open the pack of chips, or biscuits, or whatever the

hell it is you're munching on, and you don't stop munching until they're all gone (and sometimes it can even be a surprise to you when you reach the bottom of the empty packet). This is one case where paying attention to your food will help. Again, it's worth repeating; don't eat when you're doing something else. Don't eat while you're watching TV or reading. Eat when you're fully paying attention to eating. Eat only when you're in your dedicated eating area, somewhere that lets you fully engage with what (and how much) you're eating. That way, you won't be distracted by all of the other things that you do to make yourself forget that you're gorging your face with masses of food that you don't need (or even want).

Another time that you might need to pay more attention is when you're making your meals. Sometimes you can be adding excess calories to your food without even realising; "I'm gonna be really good, and have a nice healthy salad, because salad has hardly any calories whatsoever. I'll just drizzle a bit of healthy olive oil on top, to give it some depth of flavour." That's all well and good, but 1 tablespoon of olive oil actually contains about 120 calories. Same if you've spread a tablespoon-sized amount of butter on your nice healthy brown bread sandwich, that's an extra 120 calories. A tablespoon of mayonnaise contains about 100 calories... All of these foods (yes, condiments are foods too) can cause your calories to stack up.

Note: When it comes to oils/spreads, you are still better off using olive oil and real butter than the low-fat alternatives. Margarine and all of those artificial trans-fat products are like the "sweeteners" of the fat-world, and (apparently) much worse for you than the real thing. So, stick with the real deal, but just remember to go sparingly!

So, like I said, pay attention *whilst* you're eating, but also pay attention to *what* you're eating. If you're having a nice healthy bolognaise with whole wheat spaghetti, and then you dump a load of cheese on top, just remember there's 110 calories in quarter of a cup of shredded mild cheddar cheese. If you're having a roast dinner, and you grab an extra roast potato (a prime example of the carb/fat ratio), remember that a medium roast potato has about 160 calories. Sometimes we do these things without realising that we're actually putting a huge amount of extra calories into our body, and then we wonder how we miraculously got fat... well, now you know.

Do you need a full meal?
Sometimes you'll be really hungry. Sometimes you will have earned a meal. Sometimes you'll need to sit down with your family/friends/cats for a meal, and that's all fine, but if you don't *need* a full meal, then don't have one. Just have a snack instead. Let's say it's breakfast time and you're not feeling particularly hungry... Are you gonna have a huge bacon and egg roll, or could you get by with just a banana? It's lunch

time on Sunday, and you're not even thinking about food after breakfast, so would a glass of water do, or do you need to stuff down a full roast dinner just because everyone else is having it? Again, it comes back to the point of listening to your body. If your body isn't hungry, don't eat. Be smart, listen to you.

A word on gluttony (for those who feel it's relevant)
If you're a good Christian, yet you're fat, gluttony is a sin, so you're going to Hell already (right? lol). In all seriousness though, what's your excuse for gluttony? Why do you have to have the large pizza, fries and a six pack, instead of just a small pizza and a beer or two? What's making you buy the triple pack of chocolate cookies, instead of just the single pack, or a couple of individual cookies? If you want to stop being a fat ass, then you're gonna have to stop acting like a fat ass... So, either do it, or start saving up your money for a motorised mobility scooter to drag your fat ass round the supermarket to pick up your XXXL pizza and your football-team-sized pack of cookies and a loooong stick to use to wipe your ass with when you can no longer reach it!
#WowThatEscalatedQuickly

Again, it comes down to the fact that you need to think about your choices and be accountable for them. *You* are in control of your life, not me, not good ol' Jesus Christ or Allah or Buddha or Ronald Mc Fucking Donald. You are accountable for your actions, not your friends and family, YOU. If your willpower is so lacking that you feel you can't control your gluttony or your cravings, then go find someone who can help you. A dietician, a personal trainer, a hypnotherapist, a counsellor or psychologist, whatever you have to do to get yourself to the stage where you can be accountable for your actions, do it. Or do your fast, and then go to McDonalds and have 10 double cheeseburgers (and a diet coke) and wonder why you're making no progress. #Derp

What's on the menu?
Some people work a lot better, smarter and healthier if they have a plan of action – in this case it's a meal plan. You can set up your daily meals on a chart, so that you know what to eat and when. It's not for everyone, but for some people this simple idea is enough to completely fix decades of sloppy eating habits. Even if you just write down a weekly plan of what your "main meal" every day is going to be, that can stop you from thinking "hmmm, I don't know what to have, maybe I'll just order a takeaway so I don't have to decide".

Making decisions is a good thing, it is character building, so if planning your meals in advance will stop you from having a brain-fart and ordering a large takeaway pizza (and probably eating all 2,500+ calories-worth), then maybe it's time to start creating your own personal menu each week. Capeesh? #IKnowItsSpelledCapisce #SomePeopleCanOnlyReadPhoneticallyTho

Calorie counting

Unless you're a pro athlete and you need to be a certain bodyweight, or you're a bodybuilder/actor and you need to strip down to a single-digit body fat percentage before you step on stage or in front of a camera, odds are you probably don't need to count your calories *every* day. Obviously if you're doing the 50% Plan or The Weekender Plan, you'll need to be able to figure out what constitutes 500/600 calories of food, but that's pretty easy to do, so don't worry *too much* about it.

Some people, however, really enjoy calorie counting, so if you're the type of person that does, and you want to monitor your calorie intake and your "macros" (macronutrients; protein/carbs/fat), then you can get awesome apps that will help you do just that. Search for "calorie counting apps", read the reviews and pick the one that works best for you. These apps save a load of time, because they do all the calculations for you, all you've gotta do is input the type/amount of food you're eating. If you're going to eat the same meals over and over, you can even input those combinations, and one meal = one click. It's so easy, even Kanye could do it. #GoWest

There are also some websites out there that will calculate exactly how many calories someone of your age/weight/activity-level should be consuming, and the ideal breakdown of macronutrients you should be aiming for. Google "macros calculator" or "IIFYM" and it should bring up some options for you. But like I said, unless you're a bodybuilder, you probably won't need to bother with these. It can get a little complex and convoluted, and this book is here to make things simple!

How to eat well
As previously mentioned, you ideally want to be eating real food, i.e. natural food, i.e. not processed crap. You'll be able to eat more volume of food for less calories (remember the fries/cucumber comparison earlier?) and by eating healthier food, you'll get more vitamins and nutrients. You'll feel healthier, you'll feel fuller for longer, your body will be able to more easily process your food, and obviously you should lose weight!

I'm not giving you any pre-designed "set meal plans" and menus. I'm also not gonna list a whole bunch of foods and their calorie contents. I do, however, urge you to read the labels of the food you're eating, because they will tell you how many calories are in what. Even fast food joints should be doing this too, and if they don't, you should be able to look online to find out what excessive amounts of calories are contained in whatever monstrosity they're serving up. You won't have to do this for too long however, because it soon becomes something you can pretty much accurately estimate (with your eyeballs), and you'll soon begin to realise what types of food are best/worst for your waistband.

I'm going to repeat the key take-home point of this section again, just to make sure that this highly-useful nugget of information sticks in your head:

Make yourself aware of how many calories you are putting into your body!

If you want to lose weight, this is often the #1 factor. Maybe you're consuming 4000+ calories a day by eating the wrong kinds of foods (and drinks), but you might not even realise it... Well, it's time to be responsible for your choices and realise what you're putting into your body! Like I said, you don't need to do full-on calorie counting, logging every morsel of food every time you eat, but it's a good idea to know how many calories are in the foods (and portion sizes) that you *are* eating, just so you know whether you're being excessive or not. Read the labels. Do a little research. It doesn't take long, and it can be very enlightening (and sometimes surprising)!

Food choices
I told you I'm not giving you a meal plan, and I'm not but, because I'm a kind and considerate author, here are a few brief suggestions about types of healthier meals you could go for...

Note: I am not a chef, so you're gonna have to figure out the recipes for yourself. #GoogleIt

Stew, curry, chilli, bolognaise, all of those kinds of things are awesome, because you can bulk them out with a load of vegetables, you can stick some nice lean meat in there, chicken, beef, lamb, whatever, and they taste great! You don't even need to have pasta/rice/potatoes with them if you don't want to, just stick more vegetables in! That'll fill you right up, and because you've got a (relatively-healthy) sauce with them, it won't just taste like bland vegetables, it'll taste absolutely delicious (and way better than processed crap)!

You can buy pre-made sauce mixes from the supermarket if you want to, but you can actually make super low-calorie home-made versions, which often taste just as good. You can make a basic (and pretty tasty) curry sauce just using milk and curry powder. Bolognaise sauce is practically just a can of diced tomatoes and some herbs. A lot of the time, simple sauces are just as good, and you can save money that way too ...and who doesn't love money! Hippies, that's right. #Don'tBeAHippy

Soup. Soup is amazing. Boil your favourite vegetables, maybe add some meat, blend it up with some water and BOOM, you got soup. It ain't rocket-science! The combinations of soup you can make are extensive, and it can be good to experiment with different combos. Soup is a great way to get nutrients and it can be super filling too!

When you're making soup, stews, and other saucy foods, a great thing to do is make huge industrial-sized batches, and then freeze down portions, so that you don't have to cook a new meal every day of the week. You can just open up the freezer, grab a container and re-heat it! Obviously, you might need a decent sized freezer if you're doing more than one "batch-freeze", but once it's done, it can stay frozen for weeks/months. Now that's efficient!

Note: If you re-heat frozen meals, obviously make sure they're properly re-heated, and well-cooked all the way through. Especially with poultry and pork, as you don't wanna make yourself sick! Make sure that the food is boiling hot all the way through*.

* Disclaimer: Contents will be hot... lol

Salads are healthy. DUH! Like, obviously! Everyone knows salads are generally a healthy option (well, depending on whether or not you slop a load of salad-dressing/mayo/oil on top, that is). I find that a great way to brighten up a dull salad, is to add a huge slab of meat to it, because meat is great! #IDontLikeSalad #AllAboutThatProtein #SideSalad4Life

Meat and veg (not meat and 2 veg) is simple, effective and delicious. Add some good-carbs if you want to bulk it out a bit (but remember to go easy on the carbs). Steak, broccoli and sweet potato... delish!

Chicken, peas and a bit of brown rice... yum! Tuna, sweetcorn and brown pasta... damn tasty! Stir fried vegetables with king prawns, garlic, ginger and a little chilli sauce... holy moly, that's a mouth-gasm! Like I said, there are tons of things you can do with healthy food, you also have the internet! Recipe websites are a dime a dozen (if you manage to navigate to them without being side-tracked) so there's no excuse to pretend like you can't cook some simple, healthy, tasty food!

Note: If you're being really strict with what you're eating, you'll come to really love and appreciate herbs, spices and seasoning, because a bit of seasoning done right can turn a dull meal into some gourmet-style shit! #RorysOffensiveFoodTips

Now, onto snacks! How about a handful of nuts, a piece of meat (oh yis), pickled onions, a vegetable (raw carrots are great), a celery stick with a bit of peanut butter or cream cheese, a piece of fruit or a protein shake/bar (good for gym rats, but also a great snack for "normals" too) ...and not forgetting our trusty pal water, a great 0-calorie way to fill you up until your next proper meal! You must remember; a snack is meant to be a snack (which generally means it's meant to be small and light). If you're eating a whole 200g/7oz family bag of tortilla chips as a snack, that's almost 1000 calories, i.e. that's almost half of your daily recommended calorie intake, and I got sour news for ya Jack... that ain't a snack! So, snack appropriately, or maybe, just maybe, you could wait until your next meal before choosing to shove any more food into your body! You're not going to starve to death by doing this, and you may find you appreciate your meals even more!

A final point; some people like to chew sugar-free gum rather than snack, and though it's a nice idea in theory (it's something to do with your mouth that doesn't pack on the pounds), by chewing gum you begin to salivate, which means your body may begin to expect food... Again, the same as with the diet sodas, etc. tricking your body with sugar-free shit, or the expectation of food is apparently not too good for your insides. That said, I'm not telling you *not* to do it, it's your choice (and it *is* allowed while fasting)!

Note: Sugar-free gum can also be a good solution to "keto breath" (bad breath which can *occasionally* happen with fasting, as well as with other "ketogenic" diets ...it's not that common though).

What's for breakfast?
Break-fast is whatever meal you have, directly after your fast. Depending on your schedule, it could be anything, it doesn't have to be a traditional breakfast food. Whatever your break-fast food is, it can be a good idea to have it ready to go (especially if you break your fast when you're not at home), because there are all too many unhealthy, tempting options available for us, and by the end of a fast you could

possibly be more inclined to grab the first delicious-looking/smelling thing that you come into contact with. If you have something delicious and healthy with you, however, then you can stay on track and feel good in the knowledge that you are in control of your life, your eating habits and your constantly improving body shape! #BreakfastOfChampions

But what about restaurants?
As naturally social creatures, human beings often want to sit around a table, watching each other eat. Pretty weird when you think about it but, hey, it's a part of most of our lives. If you're on an alternate-day plan and an event falls on a fast day, you have two options; order the smallest thing on the menu (i.e. around 600 calories-worth) or "fuck it" and just eat. There's no way around that so, yet again, your choices are all down to you, your goals, resolve and willpower. As mentioned before, if you're required/choose to eat out a couple of times a week, and you choose to "fuck it" every time, then you're not gonna lose weight, so you may want to re-evaluate which eating plan is right for you/whether you actually want to lose weight at all!

If you only eat out irregularly, and you employ the healthy-food-choice knowledge that you've just read, then you'll pretty much be able to sail through occasions where you are required to eat out with minimal "collateral damage". TBH, even if you eat the worst thing on the menu, if you're only doing it once-in-a-blue-moon, then it's not gonna be that detrimental to your progress. If, however, you're doing a Morgan Spurlock (Google: "Super Size Me"), and eating at fast-food joints every day, then you'd best come to terms with your weight and buy yourself a bunch of pregnancy pants to wear. #ComfyAsFuck #FatshionStatement

How to Exercise

You've reached the last section of the book. So, now you know exactly what to eat (or not eat) for better success, let's take it one step further and talk about physically moving your body in order to burn fat! Yes, I'm talking about exercise. Exercise comes in all shapes and sizes, and there are thousands of books on the subject, so I'm not going to go into too much depth, because quite frankly if you're fairly overweight, the best thing that you can do alongside your fasting plan (and monitoring your food intake), is to actually get your ass moving. You don't need to know complex exercise routines, just get out and exert yourself a bit more than you have been doing and then you can progress from there! Exercise can help us live longer, boost our immune systems, boost our confidence, not to mention make us faster, stronger, leaner and more awesome in general!

Why exercise sucks for weight loss
Yeah, you read that right. There are numerous reasons why exercise often won't work (by itself) to help people lose weight, the number one reason being: You can't out-exercise a bad diet! If you're very fat, there's a very high chance that you're probably not gonna be running on the treadmill non-stop for an hour. Even if you *did* manage to do that you'd probably over-estimate how many calories you'd burn in that amount of time…

If you're about 16 stone (or 224lbs/102kg), and you ran non-stop at a speed of 5mph, which is like running a mile every 12 minutes, you'd burn a total of *around* 800 calories in an hour (in fast food terms, that's pretty much a big mac and regular fries). So, considering a pound of human fat contains about 3,500 calories, that means you'd have to run non-stop at that speed for over 4 hours to shift just 1lb. Now sure, if you add in some exercise whilst continuing to eat crap like normal, you won't gain *as much* weight as you normally would... but you probably wouldn't lose much either.

There's another common mistake that can screw up your exercise-related weight loss... Sometimes when people do an awesome workout, and burn hundreds and hundreds of calories, they then feel that because they've had a great workout and worked really hard that they deserve a reward! The problem is, by working your ass off for an hour, and then going home and eating a huge bar of chocolate or drinking a bottle of wine (or whatever "reward" you choose), you're pretty much just making work for yourself for no reason. It'd be much easier to *not* run and to *not* have the reward (and you'd probably get very similar results). #Logic101

So, what's the point then?
Well, the point is to work on your self-discipline. If you're reading this book, odds are high that you're already eating more food than your body needs for

energy, and not moving around enough. That's generally why people get fat. So, if you choose to exercise, also make the choice to either keep your calorie intake the same, or (preferably) less than normal. This will mean, rather than using your daily calories to make more fat, your body will instead use them as fuel for when you exercise, to help build muscle, and to help you recover. Adding excess calories on top of what you normally eat will stop this from happening (or slow the process).

Our brains have evolved to automatically remind us that if we've been exercising (or exerting ourselves) for a long period of time, then we should probably stop or refuel. This means that generally after a bit of exercise, your body will try and make you feel tired and hungry. The feeling of tiredness is intended to stop you from "wasting" more energy. The feeling of hunger... well, you get the idea. The thing is, your brain (the primal, animal part of it) doesn't *know* that you are guaranteed to get rest later, it doesn't *know* your next meal is a sure thing. But you *do* know that, so you have the option to override your primal mind, because in this case, you know better! Yeah, sometimes it'll take a bit of willpower but, hey, if you want results then I'm sure you'll be fine with that!

Ain't nobody got time fo' dat!
Exercising takes time, that's a fact, but so does stuffing your face with meatballs and gin. So does watching movies and TV shows, reading books, going

out with friends, procrastinating on Facebook, YouTube, Twitter, Instagram, 9gag, Grinder or whatever other online places you might spend too much time "exploring". A *good* workout can be over and done with in just 15 minutes, and you have a whopping 1,440 minutes a day. So, be brutally honest with yourself...do you *really* not have time?

Sure, there can be things that increase your workout time, such as; going to the gym, waiting for equipment, showering, etc. but you don't *have* to go to the gym to exercise. It's not mandatory. If you're just starting out, and if you're pretty overweight, you might want to start with the basics...

Start off easy
Some people like to go into a new routine of exercise with all guns blazing, and though that might seem like a good idea, it could have the reverse effect. If you start off too fast/heavy/long you could easily do yourself an injury, as your body probably isn't used to doing exercise yet. So, treat your body like an exercise-virgin; start off slow and steady until it gets used to the moves, and then when it feels right, you can start to go harder, faster and for longer (lol).

Also remember, as a beginner you probably don't need to exercise for any more than an hour, max! Honestly, if you can go for longer than an hour, you're probably not working hard enough during that time. Exercising for over an hour can also reduce testosterone levels (in both men *and* women), which can zap your energy and screw up your mood too.

How to exercise effectively

With many *uneducated* overweight people at the gym, the exercise of choice is often a slow (and I mean slow) walk on a treadmill, followed by flopping a couple of those flimsy pink dumbbells around aimlessly. They do this day in, day out, making barely any progress, and then they quit, thinking; "Well, I thought going to the gym was meant to help me lose weight". Let me put it to you like this; if you went to school and sat at the back of the class, looking out the window, daydreaming and never listening to a word the teacher said, would you expect to pass the final exam? No. The act of *going to school* does not equal learning, if it did, we wouldn't need exams, because we'd all have learnt exactly the same stuff by osmosis or something. The same goes for the gym. If you go to the gym expecting to get fit just by *being there*, without putting in any effort, well, you're gonna have a baaaad time.

Luckily, now you know that a gym membership alone won't help you towards your goal, and that you have to be willing to put in some effort, to challenge yourself and to commit to working for the end result. If you choose to do a certain exercise (walking for example), then you will need to begin to push yourself (safely) as it becomes appropriate. Walking at the same slow speed can be a great starting point, but in the *long-term*, you'll need to make it more challenging, otherwise your results will plateau (stop) and you'll get bored and quit. How will you make it more challenging? Well, you can start to walk faster, you can walk on an incline, you can even walk carrying extra weight. There are plenty of options, but you've just gotta keep in mind that your fitness and your abilities *will* improve with time and experience, so you *will* have to continuously push your limits (as uncomfortable or daunting as that may sound right now – it'll be worth it, trust me).

But it's just not "me"
FYI, you don't have to be a "certain type of person" to exercise. I used to be a couch potato, mega-lazy. I would stay glued to the TV or computer for hours/ days on end. Exercise was not something I ever chose to do. I was bad at sports in school, and as a child, I would always choose to stay inside while my friends went out to play. To me, exercise sounded like a lot of hard work for no reason. As it turns out, however, there is a reason... Exercise makes you feel amazing! It seriously does, and not only from the release of feel-good chemicals (endorphins) you get when you exercise, but also, from the feelings of accomplishment, achievement and self-confidence you get when you start to push yourself further than you ever imagined you could go. If my lazy 18-year-old self could've seen into the future, seeing how I look now (and seeing that I exercise), he'd probably have an existential crisis! Which is pretty cool.

Exercise: Cardio

So, let's start off with cardio (cardiovascular exercise). Cardio is any type of *aerobic* exercise (meaning it will improve the efficiency of your body at using oxygen). These exercises are generally "rhythmic", continuous and use large muscle groups.

Note: You may want to check with your doctor/ physician before taking part in any exercise, and if any exercise causes you physical pain, you should not continue, or should replace the exercise with another that doesn't negatively affect you (...if exercising is just a little bit uncomfortable however, that doesn't count).

For those who like to sit: Walking

Walking is a great place to start. It's low impact, you (hopefully) don't need a lesson on how to do it, and you don't need a gym membership either! Walk out your front door and then keep going. Walking on flat ground at a moderate pace doesn't burn masses of calories, but if you live a highly sedentary lifestyle (i.e. you barely ever move your body if you can help it), it's the logical choice to start off with. Walk as much as you can comfortably (or uncomfortably) manage – the amount you can manage will increase pretty quickly if you stick with it and do it every day. Also, as with most of these cardio options, the more excess fat and weight you lose, the easier and more comfortable the exercises are going to get!

When walking gets easier, walk a bit faster, walk a bit further, walk on inclines, stick a weighted backpack on – these are all great ways to get more out of walking. If you're walking on a treadmill, don't hold on to the rails! By holding on to the rails, you're reducing the amount of forward momentum that you need to produce with your legs – this defies the point of being on the treadmill. Use your legs, and if it's too fast, then turn the speed down a little bit until you can *just* handle it. Don't turn it down to the point that it becomes easy, if you're not getting tired/sweating after 5 minutes, you're probably not going fast enough. #GoHardOrGoHome

Take it to the next level (literally): Stairs
Use your skills at walking to move your body up and down sets of stairs. You don't need a Stairmaster machine to do this, just find a set of stairs in/near your home and walk up and down them. Do it more than once. See how many times you can go up and down the stairs without stopping. Sure, if you're in public people might wonder what the hell you're doing, but who cares? If you *are* bothered by looking out of place, then you can always get yourself a gym membership so you can get sweaty on the stair machine in a room full of people doing the same thing. Stairs are great and are a step up from walking (no pun intended). You'll burn almost double the number of calories walking up and down stairs than you would if you were just walking.

Note: Escalators don't count.

Run, Forrest, run: Jogging/Running/Sprinting
Running is running. You can run fast or slow. Slow
running becomes jogging, fast running becomes
sprinting. Again, it ain't rocket science; one foot in
front of the other, and repeat. You can run on a
treadmill, through the park, along the street, on the
beach (if you like a challenge). You can run for long
periods of time, marathon-style, or you can do
sprinting (running at 100% exertion) for short bursts,
kind of like interval training (which we'll cover in a
while). If you're going to run, I highly recommend
investing in a decent pair of running shoes, or at
least something with a bit more support than regular
trainers/sneakers (just thinking of your health and
wellbeing here).

Running is the logical progression when you find that
walking (fast) isn't doing enough for you anymore.
Similar to walking, if you want to make running
harder (read: more effective), stick a weighted
backpack on, run faster, run further, run up and
down hills. Again, if you're running on a treadmill,
remember that holding the rails is cheating (and also
if you're running at a decent pace, it makes it a lot
less safe), so don't do it!

On your bike: Cycling
Cycling is a great, low-impact exercise, and it's
usually good for people that struggle to walk/run due

to knee problems (though sometimes it can be exactly the opposite, so be aware of what your body is telling you). Sure, you need equipment for this; you have the option of getting an actual bike, a stationary bike/exercise bike, or a gym membership (if your gym of choice doesn't have an exercise bike, choose another gym). Obviously, to buy a good bike can be expensive, and to buy a good stationary bike can sometimes be even more expensive, but you can pick up second-hand/used models in the classifieds or on eBay for next to nothing, and generally they'll do the job.

If you get an actual bike, you can cycle a long way in one direction and then come back, or you can do circuits/laps, whichever appeals to you more. If you want to make cycling harder, then cycle faster and use inclines if possible. The stationary machines that you'll find at the gym have different pre-set programs that you can use, or you can set it manually to a certain level of resistance. For fat-loss purposes, stationary bikes are pretty much just as good as the "real thing".

Get moist: Swimming
Swimming is another great choice of cardio for people who have joint problems, as swimming tends to be a lot easier on the joints than other types of exercise. When I say swimming, I don't mean lazing around in the shallow end blowing bubbles out of your shorts, I mean doing lengths of a pool (or in a

natural water source, if you're a competent swimmer and feel you can do it safely). Swimming tends to burn slightly less calories than running, but at the same time, it's still a really good calorie burner and you're pretty much involving your entire body, so you're getting all the muscles working, which is great!

Don't like anything so far? Try the Cross Trainer
Generally, you're only gonna find a cross trainer machine worth using at the gym, the ones you can buy for home use generally aren't that great (unless you go for the gym-standard, expensive models). Cross trainers use upper and lower body and offer a pretty good workout (even if you mostly see women on these machines at the gym, they're good for men too #EqualGymRights). These machines are fairly good on the joints, so another good option if walking/ running/cycling/etc. doesn't work for you. This machine uses an elliptical range of motion for the legs, meaning you swing them backwards and forwards in an arc/oval (depending on the machine), whilst pumping the handles backwards and forwards with your arms at the same time. Sounds easy? Trust me, it's not, especially when you up the resistance!

Row, row, row your boat!
Rowing is an awesome form of cardio, mainly involving the upper body. Rowing machines can be fairly pricy, so a gym might be your best option (unless you've got your own rowing-boat moored at

your private dock). It sounds like it would be easy (as you get to sit down), but don't let appearances deceive you, rowing can be hard. As such, it's very effective for fat burning ...if you can keep it up!

Skipping/Jump Rope; it's not just for kids
If running for an hour burns 800 calories, skipping for an hour would burn more like 1,300... Skipping is hard work, but luckily that means less time working out (which is always nice). Grab a rope, hold an end in each hand, jump over it, swing it back over your head, repeat until you vomit (kidding... but it's worth noting that sometimes if you seriously overdo exercise/push your personal limits too far, you can actually make yourself sick, especially when doing high-intensity stuff). #VomTastic

You don't have to skip with a rope, you can just jump up in the air continuously, but the rope is good incentive and it makes you jump at the right pace, whereas if you're just jumping, you can slack off easier. Just remember, this type of exercise is super high impact, and if you're not used to it (and even if you are) you could easily cause yourself an injury. Pay attention to what your body is telling you.

Jump around...
Yes, more jumping. It's easy in principle, but there are many different ways you can do it. Here are a few of them:

Jumping jacks/Star jumps

Jump up, and as soon as you're off the floor you then need to move your legs out sideways (so you'll land with your feet further than shoulder-width apart), whilst lifting your arms sideways in an arc until they're over your head. Then jump again and move your arms and legs back to the starting position before you land. Do that over and over. Simple but effective!

Tuck jump

Jump in the air, tuck your legs into your chest, untuck, land and repeat. Pretty obvious, but make sure you untuck before you land, lol.

Box jump

Jump onto a box. Jump off it again. Repeat.

Yup.

If you wanna make this one harder, jump onto a higher box/platform. Remember to use something sturdy, because if it wobbles/collapses, you might injure yourself. Also, beware of bashing your shins and stacking it face first into the floor. That's no fun!

Squat jump

Again, pretty self-explanatory. Squat down, explosively jump up, land and immediately squat back down again, repeat. If that's too easy, you're gonna want to move on to the next one, which is:

Burpees

They sound gross, and they suck. If you've ever done burpees, you'll know how horrible they are. You'll also know that they're a super effective high intensity workout choice. To do a burpee you don't need any equipment, all you have to do is:

- Squat down
- Put your hands on the floor & kick your feet back into a push up position (squat thrust)
- Do a push up
- Keeping your hands on the floor, jump your legs back into squat position
- Explosively jump into the air, as high as possible, reaching upwards
- Land and squat down
- Repeat

Have fun! *Shudders*

Mountain climbers

This is another awesome, equipment-free exercise you can do wherever you want. For this one, you basically get into a push up position and try to knee yourself in the chest repeatedly. Sounds like fun, right? For full instructions on how to do this one, Google: "Mountain Climber Exercise Video" because that'll make much more sense than me trying to explain it here in text-form. You'll see why when you watch the video, lol.

Shadow boxing/Boxing
Shadow boxing is a great form of cardio, and it's a lot easier on the joints than actually hitting something, but hey, if you want to do that instead, that's fine too. Most decent gyms will have a punch bag, and if they don't, you can buy them pretty cheap – just make sure you learn to punch properly before you begin. Broken wrists/fingers aren't a lot of fun!

Exercise clubs and classes
There are various types of clubs and classes that you can join. You can use them if you want support, or so that you have someone to "work out" with. You could also join one that isn't for specifically for exercise/working out, such as a dancing class.

Dancing isn't exercise as you'd generally think of it, but many types of dancing are physically demanding. Obviously, you'd need to do enough of it (duration) to really get the blood pumping and, ideally, you'll want to do it *at least every other day.* Once or twice a week won't really cut it, especially if it's your only form of exercise.

There are, however, plenty of other clubs to choose from, such as; running, swimming, cycling, spinning (if you're a maniac), Zumba, Pilates, yoga, Tai Chi, bodyweight calisthenics, gymnastics, boxing, martial arts, boot camps, and the list goes on... So, if socialising and support is your thing (or even if it isn't), an exercise group can be a great idea!

Fuck it!
No, I don't mean a "fuck it" moment I mean actually go and get laid. Sex is a great form of cardio, so long as you get on top! Not to mention; sex is awesome, why wouldn't you wanna do more of it?! So, if you have the opportunity, get on with it! Go and screw your brains out, you have my blessing! lol

Note: By getting better at cardio in general, you may notice your "sexual prowess" increases too, mainly because you won't get so knackered during the act. #SexyGainz #DoSomeCockPushupsToo

HIIT/High Intensity Interval Training
I mentioned earlier about interval training, and it's a spectacular way to burn more calories and dramatically reduce your workout time. The only problem is, it suuuuuucks! The basic principle is; instead of slogging away for an hour on the treadmill at a continuous moderate intensity/pace, instead, you do just 15 20 minutes. You split this time into short sections of high intensity and low intensity, hence "intervals". So, this basically means you "sprint" as hard as you can for 30-60 seconds, then you walk/jog for the next minute, then back to sprinting, and you continue alternating these intervals until you literally want to die. If you see someone puking in the gym, odds are pretty high that they've been doing interval training! Hey, no one said all of these options were going to be easy or pretty. #TheSweatierTheBetter

I mentioned "sprinting", but with HIIT this doesn't just mean running. You can do HIIT sprints on any piece of cardio equipment (running, cycling, rowing, cross trainer, stair machine, and even swimming... but maybe stick to the first 5 unless you fancy drowning). Usually, for a beginner or someone of low-fitness, you'll probably manage 2 or 3 high intensity intervals before you want to vomit/die (assuming you push yourself). In all seriousness, you'll probably suck at doing HIIT when you start off, but don't worry, because you *will* get better at it.

When I started out doing HIIT, my first ever workout was intervals of walking vs. jogging (not even fast enough to be classified as a run), and after 3 minutes of 30-second intervals, I stopped, stumbled to the waste bin in the gym and puked my guts up (yes, gross, I know) ...but I didn't quit. I kept going back and doing HIIT, and within 3 weeks I got up to 15 minutes of intervals and had progressed from walk/jog to jog/run... (and I didn't puke any more after the first time either) ...so, you *will* improve if you stick with it. #EmbraceTheSuck

Interval training will send your pulse rate skyrocketing, and this is really good for boosting your metabolism and burning fat. Another awesome benefit is; this continues to happen *after* you finish working out. Yes, you continue burning calories even after you've left the gym, in fact the effects of interval training can continue for up to two hours after you've stopped working out – talk about bang for your buck!

If you're not experienced with cardio, it might not be a good idea to go in and try and sprint like an Olympian on your first go. You can always do as I did and start off with intervals that are challenging enough for *you*, but not over the top. Rather than doing 1-minute intervals, perhaps start off with 30 seconds or, if that's too much, start off with 15 seconds high intensity and 30 seconds low intensity. Make sure the high intensity part isn't too high (you can always increase it later on), and that the low intensity isn't too low (it needs to be a lot easier, but not a snail's pace! You need to keep moving).

A final point; interval training is also great if you're looking to build muscle. Whereas regular (steady state) cardio can burn fat *and* muscle, interval training tends to just burn fat. This is ideal if you don't wanna sacrifice your "gains" (i.e. muscle), but you still wanna get lean and ripped!

Exercise: Resistance training/weight lifting
As mentioned, cardio is generally good for burning fat, but as a rule it sucks for building muscle (unless of course you're doing sprints/HIIT, which can potentially help to build a little bit). If you do want to build your muscles, then you'll need to engage in some kind of resistance training program. Now, you might think you'd have to go to a gym for this, but

actually, it's not mandatory! Unless you're wanting to look like a pro bodybuilder (i.e. with monstrously huge muscles) or get as strong as an Olympic lifter, then you don't need to go overboard with your workouts. You can even do them at home if you'd prefer. Here's how:

Calisthenics
Calisthenics are body-weight/resistance training exercises that do not require equipment (or only the most basic things, like a pull up bar). If you'd like to build a bit of muscle, calisthenics would be a logical starting point. I'm not going to go into too much detail, because there are hundreds of books and videos out there on body-weight workouts (try searching; "bodyweight workout routine" on YouTube… you'll be there a while). That said, here's a really simple and effective list of the types of exercises that you should probably include if you want to begin to develop the overall musculature of your entire body…

Squats, lunges and calf raises will build your leg muscles. Push ups/press ups will develop your chest and your triceps (back of your arms). Pull ups/chin ups will build your back muscles and your biceps. If you want to work your shoulders, you can do a pike push up (a push up with your body at a 90-degree angle, your feet and hands on the floor, and your butt in the air, so that you push up using your shoulders instead of your chest), and once your shoulders get stronger, handstand push ups provide a great shoulder workout. Just those exercises alone should, if done properly and consistently, set you on the road to at least a half-decent, muscular (but not *overly* muscular) physique.

Note: Whether male or female, resistance training (even "weight lifting") won't make you look "huge" or "too muscly", unless you're training (and eating) like a bodybuilder... That takes a lot of time, effort and "supplements" and doesn't just happen by lifting some light weights/doing bodyweight exercises.

Obviously, some of those exercises may be too much for you to start off with, and others may be too easy. There are variations of most of these calisthenics exercises that will either make them easier or harder. For example; pull ups may be too hard initially (especially if you're carrying a lot of extra body weight to lift), so you could start off doing table pull ups, or pull ups with your feet on a chair, to aid you. Conversely, squats may be too easy initially (but if you're overweight, I doubt it), if they are, you can work towards doing 1-legged (pistol) squats, which are much more challenging!

There are tons of books and YouTube videos out there that give you really good instructions on how to do body weight exercises and how to steadily develop your strength. I personally started with "Convict Conditioning" (the first book), which is really good, and also found "You are your own Gym" to be pretty decent, with some good instructional pictures too. #IDontGetPaidForSayingThat

Once you get stronger and more experienced, you'll be able to consider more advanced moves such as "muscle ups" (a pull up where you go above the bar, and dip back down), the "human flag" (where you hold onto a vertical pole and hold your body out horizontally) and all kinds of other challenging feats. So, like I said, you can get a *great* body without even going within 50 feet of a gym, just keep that in mind!

Weight lifting
Even though I said you don't have to go to the gym to build muscle, there's a reason why people with great physiques tend to lift weights; because it works. You don't have to go to a gym to lift weights, you can buy a set of weights that you can use at home if you'd prefer to be hidden from the eyes of other gym-goers (introverts need gains too you know). Again, you've just gotta figure out what's gonna work best for you environment-wise, equipment-wise, time-wise, social-wise and any-other-considerations-wise.

Once you've decided whether to work out at home or at the gym, you've got another choice to make. "Weight lifting" covers a really broad spectrum of possibilities, the main contenders being hypertrophy training/bodybuilding (building big muscles), strength training/power lifting (building strength) and (forgive me) "CrossFit" (building functional strength, endurance and flexibility). The "free weights" (i.e. dumbbells, barbells and kettlebells) and "resistance machines" in the gym can *all* be utilised, whatever your end goal (size/strength/conditioning), but it's *how* you use them that determines how your body will respond to the input. So, here's a basic rule of thumb with regards to "reps" vs. weight:

Note: A "rep" (repetition) is doing 1 of whatever exercise you're doing. A "set" is the total number of reps you do in one go. If you do a set of 8 push ups, you'll have done 8 reps.

Low reps (1-6) + Heavy weight
= Strength gains

Moderate reps (7-12) + Moderate weight
− Muscle size gains

High reps (13+) + Light weight
= Conditioning/Endurance (...up for debate)

That basically means, lift heavier weight for less repetitions and you'll get stronger. Lower the weight a little, up the repetitions a bit and you'll build bigger muscles. Some people believe that doing really high repetitions with really low weight will burn more fat, but the jury's out on that one. Personally, I'd advise you to stick with building strength or building muscle as your main goal, because the more you work on building muscle/strength, the more fat you're going to burn naturally as your muscles develop.

Another good point to remember when it comes to sets and reps is that generally you won't just do 1 set for each exercise, bodybuilders for instance will often do something like 3 sets of 12 reps for each exercise they do. You might assume therefore that the strength trainers who do 3 sets of 5 reps would have a shorter workout than the bodybuilders, but the fact that they are lifting a much larger weight often means they need more time in between sets to recover.

You might again assume that building strength and building muscle are the same thing, but they're not. Sure, if you're building muscle you're generally going to build your strength at the same time, but the strength is more of a "side effect" of building larger muscles. The same is true of strength training, with muscles being more of a side effect, but either way, you're gonna be building some muscle.

A lot of people don't want to step on stage as a bodybuilder, or enter powerlifting competitions, most people just want to look a little bit more muscular, or maybe be a bit stronger. That's fine, and I'm going to assume that you're probably one of these people (for now).

I suggest that if you are new to the world of weightlifting, you should probably start off relatively light. Your body isn't used to moving heavy weights, and so by "jumping in at the deep end" you can injure yourself. I know this... I have done this... Now, years after injuring myself back when I first started weightlifting, I still have joint issues. I still have to wear wrist supports so I can lift without pain. I can't even do a pull up (comfortably) without my wrist wraps... Had I progressed from light weights to heavier weights gradually, I may well have avoided this pain (and trust me it's a pain, both physically, and a metaphorical pain in the ass!) but I made the mistake of "ego-lifting" or "trying to look cool to impress the girls in the gym" (lol). Long story short; highly un-recommended, so start off light. Yeah, you might "look weak" for a while, but hey, it's better to look weak and gradually progress and get stronger, than to mess yourself up from the get-go and actually end up not being able to lift at all, right?

On that note, you need to either do your research on the exercises I'm about to tell you or get yourself a personal trainer for a couple of sessions. This isn't an exercise book, so I'm just going to give you a brief list of exercises and it's up to you to learn how to do them properly and *safely*. Also, gym equipment can be dangerous (you'll learn this the first time you drop a 20kg/45lb plate on your toe or bash your head on a bar), and though it might seem like gyms are full of meatheads throwing iron around, weightlifting is actually quite a precise discipline.

You need to learn to respect the weights, and to know how to properly perform *every* exercise you're doing, unless you want to chance getting injured by just "having a go" (again, not recommended). There are so many books and places online that can show you how to do exercises properly, a great place to start is bodybuilding.com – an amazing resource for gym-goers of all shapes, sizes, disciplines and goals.

Weight lifting exercises
As mentioned, there's bodybuilding and strength training (yeah, yeah, and CrossFit too I guess). Generally, people training for strength will work on the "big 3" exercises, which are; squat, deadlift and bench press. These are "compound" movements (i.e. they use more than one muscle group) and are 3 of the main lifts that are generally featured in strength competitions. These exercises are great for strength, but also great for building muscle (if you change the reps/weight, remember!)

If you could only ever do 5 exercises, these 3 would be included. If I were to choose the final 2 exercises to add to that list, they would be the pull up/chin up and the overhead press. By doing just these 5 exercises properly and consistently, you can build a great all-round physique.

Bodybuilders, however, tend to use a greater variety of exercises, and more "isolation" exercises (using just one muscle at a time, as opposed to compound exercises that use more than one). Some do this for variation, some want to "hit the muscles from a different angle", others find that certain exercises screw with their joints (for instance, a barbell bench press might cause you pain, but if you did the same exercise with dumbbells it might not, due to the slightly different angles/range-of-motion involved).

Here's a list of popular, tried-and-tested exercises that you can do. Most of them have many variations, but you might as well stick to the good ol' originals to begin with, until you get an idea of what you should/shouldn't be doing. Some of these exercises can be done with free weights, machines and/or both. I have separated the list into body parts:

Chest (and Triceps)
Bench Press
Chest Press
Pec Fly
Cable Fly
Dips

Back (and Biceps)
Deadlift
Pull Up/Chin Up
Pull Down
Row

Shoulders
Overhead/Military Press
Front Raise   (just for front part of shoulder)
Lateral Raise (just for middle part of shoulder)
Rear-Delt Fly (just for back part of shoulder)

Traps (upper back/in between Shoulders)
Shrug
Upright Row

Legs (Quadriceps/front)
Squat
Lunge
Leg Press
Leg Extension

Legs (Hamstrings/back)
Deadlift
Leg Curl
Good Morning

Legs (Calves)
Calf Raise
Seated Calf Raise
Horizontal Calf Raise
Donkey Raise

Arms (Forearms)
Reverse Grip Curls
Wrist Roller
Wrist Curls

Arms (Biceps)
Dumbbell Curl
Barbell Curl
Hammer Curl
Concentration Curl
Cable Curl

Arms (Triceps)
Dips
Cable Pressdown/Pulldown
Overhead Dumbbell Triceps Extension
Skullcrusher
Triceps Kickback

Abs
Sit Ups
Crunches
Hanging Knee/Leg Raise
Plank

Lower back
Hyper-extensions
Good mornings

Putting them all together
There are various types of workout plan you can
choose. Some people do full body, which means you
do an exercise (or two) for every part of your body,
all in one sitting. Some people do a body split
workout, i.e. upper body one day, and lower body

the next. Some people work out one body part per day, i.e. chest one day, back the next, then legs… etc.

*Note: You can do cardio **every day**, but with weight lifting, you need to give your muscles more time to recover. Recovery is very important, and if you don't give yourself enough recovery time you could end up with injuries or getting sick.*

To start off with, aim to work out 3 times per week. I can't tell you which type of workout plan would work best for you, so you're going to have to do some research, but initially, a simple full body workout 3 times a week could be a good place to start. You could go for the 5 exercises I mentioned before or choose a selection from the list of exercises you just read, it's up to you! Just make sure whatever you do, you do it safely at a pace that's right for you. Sure, challenge yourself, but don't be silly about it!

Note: Other people at the gym don't think it's cool when you're trying to lift weights that are heavier than you can manage. Trust me, they'll know. #Don'tBeThatGuy

Remember the H^2O
I know I've said it a lot, but you've got to drink water! Keep yourself hydrated whilst exercising. You'll probably be sweating, so you're going to need to increase your intake of water to compensate for that. Even if you're not a sweaty person, you'll still

need some additional water. Remember – water is your friend. Take a bottle with you when you work out, whether cardio or weight training (also, maybe take a towel, no one likes other people's sweat on the gym equipment... that's gross).

A word on fasting for weight lifters...
Yes, you *can* exercise whilst you are actively fasting, and it *may* actually increase the fat burning effect of your workout... However, if you're doing high intensity workouts, please be aware of your energy levels. If you're going for the heaviest deadlift you can possibly manage, and you haven't eaten for 18 hours, that might negatively affect your performance. Be careful, use your brain.

If you're going to do weight lifting whilst fasting, I recommend that you get yourself some BCAAs (branched-chain amino acids). BCAAs are a great way to give your body a little fuel to stimulate protein synthesis (muscle building), but without actually having to break your fast early (as it contains no calories). I personally take 5g of BCAA powder before my workouts (and sometimes after). *If possible*, perhaps time your workout so that you break fast soon afterwards, that way your first meal goes towards refuelling and building your muscles.

Work with what you've got
We're all built differently, we've all had different things happen in our lives. Just because your friend

can run for 5 hours solid on the treadmill and feel fine after, doesn't mean you'll be able to. Just because your 85-year-old grandma can squat 400lbs raw, doesn't mean you can. We're all different, so listen to your body, learn its strengths and weaknesses and play to them. There's no point screwing yourself up before you even get started!

Sometimes things don't quite go to plan, so we might occasionally have to make a new plan, one that works for us and that we can achieve and connect with. I personally wanted to train to be super strong and to lift ridiculously heavy weights, but since I hurt my wrists, that initial goal became unlikely... Oh well, so what! Doesn't mean I quit, I just changed my plan and now I train in a different way, and I'm much stronger than I ever thought I would be... This doesn't just apply to working out either, it also applies to eating and fasting. We all have setbacks and challenges sometimes, because we all have lives. It's how you react to those challenges that matters. Some people fall down and give up, some people get up, dust themselves off and move on towards their goals in whatever ways they are able to. Know that when you want it enough, you'll always have the ability to get back up and keep going...

You can do this.

So that's it...

There you have it. You have reached the end of the book. Now all I ask is that you go out and actually do it, starting as soon as you possibly can (if you haven't already). I hope you've enjoyed reading, and that you've learned some stuff, and I'd totally appreciate it if you can take a moment to give this book a quick review on Amazon, because I would love to know what you think of it. I *personally* read all of the reviews I get, so make it honest, make it awesome!

Finally, once you've been using your plan for a while and you get some great results, I'd love to share them on the **Hypno-Fasting** website. It feels amazing to help motivate others who are just starting out on their fasting journeys. When you decide you'd like to share photos of your own transformation (before & after), visit **Hypno-Fasting.com** for instructions on how to send them in. I look forward to seeing them!

Thanks once again for reading, and now it's time for you to go and get started... Do it now... No excuses!

Rory Z Fulcher
Hypno-Fasting.com

97188994R00137

Made in the USA
Columbia, SC
07 June 2018